Also by Jane Henry Stolten, R.N.

THE HEALTH AIDE

THE GERIATRIC AIDE

HOME CARE

HOME CARE

A Guide to Family Nursing

Jane Henry Stolten, R.N.

Illustrated by Nancy Lou Gahan

LITTLE, BROWN AND COMPANY
Boston—Toronto

FIRST EDITION

T 08/75

LIBRARY OF CONGRESS CATALOGING IN PUBLICATION DATA

Stolten, Jane Henry.
  Home care.

  Includes index.
    1. Home nursing. I. Title. [DNLM: 1. Home
nursing. WY195 S875h]
RT61.S73   649.8   75-9732
ISBN 0-316-81742-2

DESIGN BY BARBARA BELL PITNOF

*Published simultaneously in Canada
by Little, Brown & Company (Canada) Limited*

PRINTED IN THE UNITED STATES OF AMERICA

To Johnny, Clarence, and Bertie,
who cared and needed care

I wish to acknowledge and thank the following sources of help and materials:

Department of Health, Education and Welfare, U.S. Government

The 1971 White House Conference on Aging

The National Health Services of Canada, Czechoslovakia, England, Hungary, and Yugoslavia

New York University Institute of Physical Medicine and Rehabilitation, New York

Visiting Nurse Service, New York

Roosevelt Hospital Home Care Service, New York

Day Hospital at the Burke Center, White Plains, New York

Martin Luther King Memorial Hospital and Health Center, New York

The Foundling Children's Center, New York

The American Cancer Society

The American Diabetes Association

The American Foundation for the Blind

To the Reader

New medical attitudes stress that, whenever possible, patients receive care at home rather than in hospitals, nursing homes, or other institutions. There are obvious advantages to home care. Patients benefit psychologically from being in the comfort, security, and status of familiar life. The costs of care are less. And treating more patients at home allows for better use of institutional space so that more patients have access to specialized treatments.

To make home care possible, many institutions now teach patients and their families how to meet special needs at home. And sometimes the fees for home care services of professional nurses or aides are covered by public health or private insurance agencies. However, family instruction is usually limited and nursing help is most often supervisory or part time. The weight of care falls on family members or friends who want to do the right things but are often confused about exactly what should be done and how to do it.

Home Care is designed to help anyone who must care for an ill or feeble person at home. It can be used as a source of nursing information, a reference for better understanding of patient care, and a guide to total care. It can also be used to review certain special care instructions. It offers a broad range of nursing knowledge, covering general care from infancy through aging and the particular care of many special conditions that are often treated at home. The subject matter is intended to complement medical care or direct nursing instruction. It is *not* intended to *replace* direct medical care or nursing instruction. Correct use of the book will improve your confidence, ability, and ease in giving care; it will increase your patient's comfort and well-being.

All the information has been adapted to care at home and is presented in everyday language, with clear explanations, step-by-step instructions, and helpful illustrations. The book is divided into three main sections. Section One considers general care and its application to adult patients. Because so much of this material is relevant for older adults, adaptations for the aged are included here rather than repeated in the special chapter on aging. Section Two contains specifics about the care of many adult conditions. Section Three is limited to infant care. While it has both general and specific material, it does not repeat information given elsewhere in the book. For example, information about taking an infant's temperature is found in Section Three, but general information about temperatures and thermometers is found in Section One. In the absence of a neuter pronoun, *he, his,* or *him* is used throughout to indicate both sexes (except, of course, when the subject matter applies only to female patients).

To use the book to best advantage, first consider your patient's overall condition. Take into account chronic problems as well as immediate ones and what the doctor has ordered for any and all conditions. For example, suppose the patient is aging, diabetic, and hard of hearing. In addition and at the moment, he has the flu. First list the doctor's orders for the immediate condition. They might be: temperature every four hours, prescription medicine every six hours, bed rest except to go to the bathroom, and so forth. Next, list what the doctor has ordered for the patient's chronic conditions. These might be: a four-legged cane, a diabetic diet, urine testing, insulin by injection in the morning, special skin care, a hearing aid, and the like. Then read the special chapters in Section Two that concern the patient's chronic problems. After that, read the first chapter, on planning patient care, and list the patient's needs such as bathing, bedmaking, toileting, food, and fluid. Now look at all of the lists and collate them into a timed program for care. If you are unsure about anything on this list, look for that subject in the Contents or in the Index.

While this book offers the best techniques developed by professionals over many years of nursing practice, it lacks the most important ingredients of any patient's care: thoughtfulness, tenderness, and love. Since all acts of nursing are demonstrations of these qualities — and these are also the basics of family and friendly relationships — patients often benefit more from care given by those held dear than that given by strangers. Providing home nursing care allows family members and friends to express concern in active, helpful ways that strengthen affection. If such a caretaker combines concern with the knowledge he or she gains from this book, pleasure can be found in the performance of skilled home care — and, most important, the patient will benefit by the best care possible.

New York, N.Y.
January 1975

Contents

To the Reader   xi

GENERAL CARE

1   Patient Care   3
2   Vital Signs   20
3   Medicine   28
4   Sleep, Rest, and Physical Therapy   40
5   Adaptive Equipment   64
6   Feeding   80
7   Handling   97
8   Bed, Bed Equipment, and Bedmaking   113
9   Bathing, Skin Care, Massage, and Grooming   124
10   Toileting   159
11   Applying Heat and Cold   180
12   Other Useful Techniques   191

CARE FOR SPECIAL CONDITIONS

13   The Aged, or Geriatric, Patient   201
14   Arthritis   211

15   Communicable Disease
        and Isolation Technique   215
16   Death and Dying   225
17   Defective Vision and Hearing   228
18   Diabetes   236
19   Fracture   242
20   Heart and Lung Disease   247
21   Mental Disorders   261
22   Stroke   266

INFANT CARE

23   Pregnancy and Hospital Delivery Care   281
24   Preparing to Give Infant Care   287
25   Handling an Infant   298
26   Bathing, Weighing, and Measuring   306
27   Dressing an Infant   314
28   Feeding an Infant   319
29   Growth and Care   335
30   Care in Unusual Conditions   345

APPENDICES

A   Health Care Glossary   359
B   Measurements   364
C   Patients' Rights   365
D   Health Services   367
E   Doctors   371
F   National Organizations   373

INDEX   377

General Care

1

Patient Care

The possibility of sickness is always present, especially in a household with young children or older adults. It is good to accept the demands of illness as being natural aspects of life and to be prepared to meet these demands. Acceptance and preparation ease the tensions that often surround illness at home, allow for better patient care and comfort, and calm the anxieties of those who must give care.

Taking care of a patient involves both mental and physical preparation for meeting immediate and chronic care needs, as explained in the Preface. Any patient care at home also requires some basic knowledge, materials, and organization, which are presented in this chapter.

Mental preparation includes considering the patient, and understanding how a doctor thinks about a patient, and how the doctor orders care. It means learning to keep a home care record or chart, to observe a patient for symptoms, to report observations, to relay information to a doctor by telephone, to be aware of a patient's safety needs, and to maintain a sanitary environment for the patient. Physical preparation involves collecting necessary materials and organizing them in the best way possible.

Three things should be considered about any patient: his body, his mind, and his emotions. These elements are so interwoven that they cannot be separated. Illness of one means illness of the others, and all must have attention. But the body, mind, and emotions of each person differ and these differences depend on many factors, including

sex and age;
the kind of illness and its severity;
the patient's general health;
his history of past illnesses and hospitalizations;
his nationality, race, religion, and income;
his disposition, habits, and personality;
his social background of relatives and friends.

Let us suppose that a doctor is taking care of three people. All of them have the mumps.

The first patient is a girl of six, one of five children of a poor family. She does not speak English and has never been away from home. Her case is very severe.

The second patient is a wealthy, excitable, educated young man who has seldom been ill. He has heard that when mumps occur in a grown man, it may cause sterility. This man has a very mild case of mumps but he does not believe that.

The third patient is a lonely woman of sixty-nine. She has a mild case of mumps but is diabetic and has a heart condition.

It is easy to see that each of these patients would require different treatment, and that the severity of the disease is not always the determining factor.

So it is very necessary to think of each person as an individual with his own separate needs. Consider these needs and adapt to meet them in every way you can.

The Doctor's Orders

A patient has two kinds of needs. First, he has the ordinary needs of any person:

body warmth
air to breathe
exercise
cleanliness
food
elimination of waste
sleep

Second, he has specific needs because of his individual illness. EXAMPLE: A person with appendicitis might need

laboratory tests to determine changes in his body;
medicine to reduce the infection;
cold applied to the abdomen to control swelling;
an operation;
if operated upon, preoperative and postoperative care.

The doctor always orders care to meet the patient's ordinary and specific needs.

The doctor orders which vital signs to take and when to take them. Vital signs are: temperature, pulse, respirations, and blood pressure. He might order

temperature every morning;
temperature, pulse, and respirations four times a day;
temperature and pulse every four hours, day and night;
blood pressure once every week;
blood pressure taken once every day while lying down, sitting, and standing.

The doctor orders the patient's activity. He would order one of the following:

complete bed rest
bed rest
out of bed (at will)
ambulatory, or walking
bathroom privileges
up in chair
full activity

The doctor orders the kind of bath the patient can have; sometimes this is understood in the order for activity.

complete bed rest: implies a bedbath and making the bed with the patient in it
bed rest: implies a partial bath and making the bed with the patient in it
out of bed, ambulatory: implies a tub bath or shower and making the bed without the patient in it
bathroom privileges: needs special order for bath or shower but making the bed without the patient in it
up in chair: needs special order for bath or shower but making the bed without the patient in it

The doctor orders the patient's diet or food. He would order one of the following diets:

regular
soft
clear liquid
full liquid
special diet

The doctor orders what the patient may require for good bowel and urine function. He might order

a laxative;
an enema;
increased fluid intake;
measure fluids taken in and urine voided.

The doctor orders a sleeping medication if necessary.

Home Care Record or Chart

Keep a record of the patient. A looseleaf notebook is good for this. Mark certain pages *Doctor's Orders* and write in any medication or treatment ordered for the patient.

Mark certain pages *Treatments*. Keep a record of the dates, times, and results of all treatments.

Mark certain pages *Temperature, Pulse and Respirations, Blood Pressure*. Keep a record of the dates, times, and amounts of these vital signs.

Mark certain pages *Daily Duties* and organize your duties.

Mark certain pages *Measured Intake and Output* (if your patient needs these) and keep an accurate record of his fluid balance. SEE: Fluid Balance.

Mark certain pages *Medications*. Keep a record of the date, time, and amount of all medicines. SEE: Medicines.

Mark certain pages *Notes on the Patient*. Keep a record of the dates and times and pertinent information about the patient's condition. EXAMPLE:

6:00 A.M. Woke up — perspiring heavily — felt weak — took
medicine.

6:30 A.M. Went back to sleep after changing pajamas and urinating — the urine was very dark yellow.

8:50 A.M. Awoke — felt much better.

9:30 A.M. Breakfast of orange juice, cream of wheat with milk and sugar, and one cup of tea — ate little cereal — drank all orange juice and tea.

10:00 A.M. Normal bowel movement — tub bath — took medicine — sat in armchair — seemed tired — said he felt cold — helped back to bed.

Such a record allows a doctor or visiting nurse to get a much more accurate picture of a patient's overall progress and needs. It should include any changes in the patient's normal behavior or ordinary needs.

Observing the Patient

Symptoms

A healthy body looks, acts, and behaves in certain expected normal ways. When sickness and aging occur, some of these ways change. Any sign of change away from or back toward normal is called a symptom.

When symptoms are confined to a small area of the body, they are called local symptoms. EXAMPLE: When skin breakdown occurs, it first shows as a reddened area.

When symptoms occur not only in the local area, but throughout the body, they are called general symptoms. EXAMPLE: A person with pneumonia would have local symptoms of cough, chest pain, difficulty in breathing, and a bloody discharge from the lungs. He would have general symptoms of an elevated temperature, a fast pulse, a feeling of extreme tiredness or collapse, changes in the color and the degree of dampness of his skin, and changes in the balance of food and fluid intake and waste outputs.

The degree and amounts of these changes would vary from time to time, so the date and the hour are as necessary to record as the symptoms themselves.

In order to diagnose and treat an illness, a doctor must know the exact location of any symptom and have a clear description of it.

EXAMPLE: Do not report that "the patient has a pain in his leg." Report in detail: "The patient has a throbbing pain in the inner side of his upper left calf. An area about the size of an orange appears somewhat swollen and is reddened. At the center of this area is a small opening in the skin, crusted with dried blood."

EXAMPLE: Do not say: "The patient has a cold." Do say: "The patient is sneezing. His nose is running, his eyes are watering, and he has a frequent wet cough."

Learn to observe and report by using all of your senses to notice changes in a patient.

See and describe:
    the general activity of a patient
    body positionings
    skin textures
    skin color changes
    the presence of discharges from any part of the body and the nature of the body's wastes: *the substance, the amount, the color, the consistency, the smell, the frequency*
    facial expressions: *eye expressions, eye changes*

Hear and describe:
    how the patient talks
    what the patient says
    how he reacts to questions
    what he leaves unsaid but indicates by actions
    noises that his body makes

Smell and describe:
    any part of the body or discharge

Touch and describe:
    any part of the body
    how the patient's body reacts to your touch

Get your patient to tell you:
    how he sees
    how he hears
    how his mouth tastes
    how he feels
    about any pain: note the following: *the exact location, the kind of pain, when it occurs, how long it lasts, if anything relieves it*
    about his mental condition through general conversation and other activities

Bathtime offers an excellent chance to observe a patient.

Sometimes there is a sudden onset of alarming symptoms that indicate the patient is in great distress. Don't panic — that's important. Do what you can for the patient in a calm, reassuring way. Get the doctor or an emergency service at once. Your behavior can mean life or death for your patient. Further, a calm attitude will control the patient's own fear and make the situation easier for him.

TELEPHONING THE DOCTOR

Before you call, have a pencil and pad ready to write down any instructions the doctor may give you. Have the patient's home chart up to date and ready for reference in case the doctor asks questions about the patient's condition.

Write down and have at hand:

1. Exactly which changes prompted you to call the doctor.
2. The time when the changes took place and how these changes differ from the patient's earlier condition.
3. What steps you took to relieve the patient.

EXAMPLE: The changes and time: "At 9:15 the patient began to breathe very fast. His pulse was fast and weak. His face was gray and sweaty. Temperature, Rectal 99.6°F. (37.5°C.). Pulse, 120. Respiration, 34."

The earlier conditions and time: "Patient's 8:00 A.M. temperature, 98.4° F. (37° C.). Pulse, 84. Respiration, 24. Patient appeared normal in every way. He was cheerful and ate all of his breakfast. He had a large soft bowel movement of dark brown stool after breakfast."

What you did for the patient's relief: "I raised the patient's head level. I started oxygen as you ordered."

After you call the doctor and reach him, his office, or his answering service, give the following information at once: "This is (*your name*), taking care of (*patient's name*) at (*patient's address and telephone number*). I am calling because of the following changes in (*patient's name*) condition."

Then give all the facts that you have written down about the changes, the earlier condition, and anything you did to relieve the patient.

Listen carefully and write down any instructions you are given by the doctor, his office, or the answering service. Ask questions if there is anything you do not understand.

Safety

Preventing Accidents

Walk, do not run.

Keep to the right side of halls and stairs.

Avoid horseplay.

Take precautions against slipping in the bathroom.

Take precautions against fires.

Avoid overwaxing floors or using scatter rugs.

Pick up or wipe up anything on the floor that does not belong there.

Do not climb on supports that are unsteady or too low to reach high things.

Do not pile things so they can topple over.

Do not leave objects where they are hidden and can be tripped over.

Keep furniture and equipment in good working condition.

Keep equipment neat and orderly to prevent injury from hidden parts.

Check linen for pins or other objects before sending it to the laundry.

Examine the electric cord and plug of any electrical equipment before use. Have frayed cords or loose plugs repaired.

Wheel, do not carry, heavy or awkward equipment.

Keep medicines, cleansers, poisons, and cleaning fluids in a safe place and plainly labeled.

Do not leave filled bottles and containers uncapped.

Be alert for unsafe conditions and do whatever is necessary to correct them.

Special Safety Measures for Patients

Special safety precautions are necessary for patients because they often suffer from conditions such as poor balance, defective vision, and mental confusion that increase the possibilities of accident.

IN BED

Use bedrails when a patient is sleeping or confused.

Do not allow a patient to get out of a high bed without help.

Do not use hot water bottles or heating pads without a doctor's order. A hot water bottle should be filled with warm water — never hot water.

Do not allow a patient to smoke in bed when alone.

Wipe the bed and mattress often with a mild antiseptic (SEE: Cleaning and Sanitizing).

Keep the bed clothing clean, orderly, and dry.

Keep the patient's belongings within easy reach.

For support, use rolled cotton blankets, sheets, or towels rather than pillows, which might cover the face and interfere with breathing.

CLOTHING AND WALKING EQUIPMENT

Be sure clothing is the correct size for the patient so that it does not interfere with his movements or cause him to trip or fumble.

Keep clothing clean and mended.

Repair shoes regularly.

See that the patient wears clothes suitable to the weather.

Be sure clothing is lightweight and does not drag on the floor or tire the patient.

Keep walking equipment in good condition and be sure that the patient uses it correctly.

HALLWAYS AND STAIRS

Be sure these areas are well lighted throughout.

Have handrails on both sides of stairs.

Have the two ends of rails shaped differently than the center portion so they can be identified by touch as well as sight.

Paint white or yellow the first and last step of a flight of stairs.

Use nonslip floor covering.

Block stairway with gate if dangerous.

BEDROOM

Cover radiators with protective frames.

Use nonslip floor covering.

Have doors open in against walls.

Use crossbars across windows with low sills.

Use sturdy, nontippable furniture.

BATHROOM

See that the patient uses an electric shaver rather than a safety razor.

Make sure that the patient uses grab rails by tub and toilet. Never let him use a towel rack as a grab rail.

Be alert for and clean floors wet with water, urine, or other fluid.

See that the room is warm and draft-free while the patient is bathing.

See that the room is well lighted.

Never use bath water hotter than 110° F. (43° C.).

Use nonslip tape and a nonslip suction pad in the tub.

FOOD

Never allow a patient to use a sharp knife or other utensil with which he can injure himself.

Use spillproof dishes and glasses if necessary.

Use unbreakable dishes and glassware if necessary.

Wash and sterilize all dishes and glassware after use.

Prepare special diets exactly as ordered.

Use a sturdy table to hold food.

Light the eating area well.

Cleaning and Sanitizing

THE BEDROOM

A patient responds well to cleanliness and order. His room should have a daily cleaning that includes the following jobs:

Check for outdated newspapers, food, dishes, used tissues, paper scraps, and remove them.

Empty the patient's wastebasket and reline it with a clean bag.

Remove articles from the tops of bedside tables and wipe the tops.

Replace articles neatly so that they are within the patient's easy reach.

Clean and refill water pitcher and glass.

Replace supplies such as tissues and drinking straws.

Dust furniture and windowsills.

Vacuum and/or mop the floor.

Straighten all furniture.

Adjust window shades, blinds, or curtains.

If the patient is confined to bed, check and clean bathing and toileting equipment and replace supplies such as soap, toilet paper, and towels.

THE BATHROOM

The patient's bathroom should have a special daily cleaning that includes the following duties:

Scrub the sink and tub with cleanser or wipe with disinfectant bathtub cleanser.

Use a toilet brush and disinfectant to scrub the inside of the toilet bowl.

Wash the outside of the toilet and the entire toilet seat with disinfectant solution.

Be sure that toilet paper is on the dispenser and an extra roll is nearby.

Clean the mirror.

Clean any other equipment.

Wipe all tiles with disinfectant solution.

Mop the floor with disinfectant solution.

Special Sanitizing of Patient's Room

This is done when a patient recovers from an illness, changes rooms, or as needed when a patient is ill over a period of several months or more.

Take all special equipment such as the washbasin, emesis basin, plastic sheeting, urinal, and bedpan to the bathroom.

TOILETING EQUIPMENT

Sanitize toileting equipment by scrubbing out; then fill to the brim with a disinfectant solution made from a household disinfectant such as Clorox (read label directions for making correct solution). Allow to soak for thirty minutes or as otherwise directed.

BASINS AND PLASTIC

Sanitize washbasins, plastic sheets, plastic pillow cases, and the like, by first cleaning them and then putting them in the bathtub to soak in a mild disinfectant solution. Follow directions given on the disinfectant container label for solution strength and time.

After sanitizing, rinse all objects, dry well, and return to patient's room or store in the Sick Care Box.

Powder plastic sheets or pillowcases to prevent their sticking together.

BED, MATTRESS, PILLOW, BEDDING

Strip bed and wash bedspread, blankets, sheets, and mattress protector. Add disinfectant or bleach during the washing. Remove mattress from bed.

Prepare a solution of disinfectant in a basin. (Wear rubber or plastic gloves to protect hands from the solution.) After dipping a clear sponge in solution, wring it as dry as possible.

If the bed is metal or another nonwooden material, wipe every part of the head, foot, legs and springs.

Wipe the mattress surface that was nearest the patient.

Put the mattress back on the bed, wiped side down.

Wipe all other exposed areas of the mattress.

Wipe the pillows with disinfectant solution.

Close the door and open the windows to air the room for as long as possible, up to twenty-four hours.

STERILIZING

Certain articles such as glasses, pitchers, and dishware should be sanitized often. This can be done by using a dishwasher or by soaking in a Clorox solution. See the label for preparation and timing instructions. Or boil dishes in a large pot with a lid and enough water to cover articles for ten to twenty minutes.

Used tissues or infectious dressings can be sterilized by burning inside a metal container in an outdoor location free of brush or other fire hazards.

Other information about sterilization can be found in Chapter 15, Communicable Disease.

Sick Care Box

It is helpful to have many of the general things needed for sick care at home together in one place. A cardboard carton plainly labeled SICK CARE can be stored in an out-of-the-way but accessible closet corner. Here are some suggestions for things to keep in this box.

FOR THE BED

plastic drawsheet (a drawsheet is an extra half sheet used under the patient to protect the bed and make changing under bed linen easier; SEE: Bedding)

plastic pillowcase cover (zippered is best)

several muslin drawsheets (these can be made from old bedsheets that have been cut in half and hemmed)

extra pillows (one adult size; one or more baby or small)

a thin cotton blanket (to be used when bathing or giving a
treatment in bed)

several large brown paper bags (to be used as bed wastebags
or to hold patient's belongings while in bed)

FOR THE BEDSIDE TABLE

a plastic cover for the tabletop

a small bell

a box of tissues

a plastic water pitcher

FOR BATHING AND GROOMING IN BED

a small standing mirror

a plastic washbasin

a soap dish

several disposable clear plastic food containers, such as are
used to package cottage cheese, in different sizes to be used
as emesis basins and sputum cups (containers to catch
vomit and spit)

a bottle of massage lotion such as Lubriderm or Vaseline Intensive Care

FOR TOILETING IN BED

a bedpan

a urinal (clean milk containers with tops removed make useful disposable urinals)

a clean disposable cloth or Handiwipe (to use as bedpan
cover)

a roll of toilet paper (storing an extra roll ensures it being on
hand)

CLOTHING

several bedgowns or old pajama tops (instructions for making
gowns are given on page 18)

RECREATION AND OCCUPATION

lightweight books and magazines

a sketch pad and colored pencils

a letter pad and envelopes, pen

a small transistor radio

fix-it equipment for small items

a sewing box for mending
small lightweight toys, coloring books, and crafts

MEDICINES
Find a special smaller box that can be kept on a high shelf out of reach of children and animals. This box is a good place to store an extra mouth or rectal thermometer and a small tube of Vaseline. During an illness the box can hold the patient's medicines.

After looking over this list, think of other useful items that your individual family members might need or like and include them in your Sick Care Box. If a patient needs special equipment, it can be obtained from a medical supply house or through your local drugstore.

Organizing Patient Care

Whenever possible the patient should have his own room and bed. However, include him in family activity as much as possible.

See that the room is clean and orderly.

Get the right bed equipment. SEE: Bed.

Position the bed in the best way for the patient. EXAMPLE: If there is danger of the patient falling out of bed, put one side of the bed against a wall and use one or more heavy chairs as rails against the exposed side. If there is no danger of falling and the patient can look out of a window if the bed is in the center of the room, put the bed there. And so on.

Supply a bedside table, preferably with a drawer and cabinet, to contain personal items such as a comb, mirror, pen and paper, and urinal or bedpan. To protect the tabletop from spills and soils, cut out a cover from a cardboard grocery box. The cover should be half an inch longer on all sides than the tabletop. Cover the cardboard cover with plastic or Contak paper.

Put a bottle or pitcher of fresh water and a drinking glass on the covered tabletop. Add a box of tissues and a small bell for summoning help. If the patient is allowed a telephone, put it here.

Line a wastebasket with a plastic bag and put it near the table within easy reach of the patient.

Supply a good light for the patient. A bed light is good, but the best is a standing lamp placed behind the table near the bed.

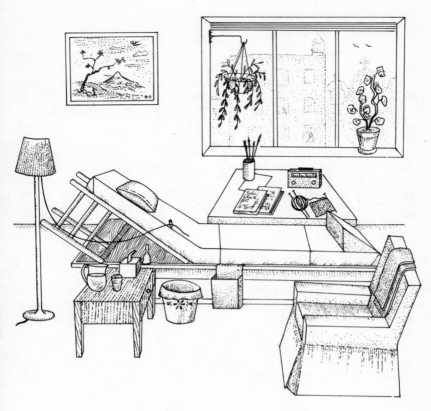

Care unit setup for a right-handed person

Extend the cord of the light switch with a string and pin a loop of the string to the undersheet of the patient's bed, or attach a remote control switch to the lamp and place the control so that it is handy for the patient when he is in bed.

Position a chair near the foot of the bed.

If the bed is high and the patient is allowed out of bed, provide a strong footstool.

Provide a table (a card table is good) within the patient's reach for recreational and occupational activities such as magazines, books, puzzles, radio, cards, and knitting. This table may also serve as a place for meal trays if the patient takes his meals in bed. A television set is good but should be used for special programs only. Whenever possible, television viewing should be with the family. SEE: Recreational Therapy and Occupational Therapy.

Provide whatever the patient may need for toileting. SEE: Toileting.

Set up a tray in the kitchen with dishes for the patient alone. Your choice would depend on the patient's interests and ability to feed himself, so they might range from the prettiest china for the able patient to special adaptive unbreakable dishware. SEE: Feeding.

Provide easy, lightweight, washable bedclothing. Plain pajama tops that open in front and tie-string pajama bottoms are usually more comfortable than other styles of night clothing. If the patient is allowed up, provide a bathrobe and slippers that give foot support. Cotton or light wool socks help keep feet warm.

Other special needs of the patient can be found in the Index under specific headings.

Making Bedgowns

The best kind of gown for the patient who must spend a great deal of time in bed is one that is comfortable, that will not easily wrinkle under his back, and that is easy to change. The gown used in hospitals is designed for these purposes. It is easy to make such gowns from men's old shirts. Simply cut off the collar and cuffs and button panels. Finish the cut surfaces with sewed-on bias tape or iron-on tape. Make tapes to tie at the neck, chest, and waist.

General Rules for All Treatments

Some rules apply to all treatments. Learn them well, for they mean greater comfort for the patient, less effort for you, and more efficient work.

Before a Treatment

Collect all the equipment for the treatment and take it to the bedside.

Wash your hands.

Tell the patient what you are going to do.

See that there are no drafts in the room.

Draw the screen or close the door.

Use a protective sheet or pad to prevent soiling or wetting the bed.

If the treatment involves the torso or the legs, fanfold the bed-clothes to the foot of the bed and cover the patient with a cotton blanket.

See that the patient is in the best position for the treatment.

During a Treatment

Watch the patient's reaction.

Stop the treatment if an unwanted reaction occurs and report to the doctor if necessary.

Stay with the patient throughout the treatment if he is giving it to himself and if his safety or emotional security demands your presence.

If you do not need to stay with the patient, see that his bell is handy before you leave.

Check on him from time to time.

After a Treatment

Replace bedclothes and patient's gown if necessary.

See that the patient is in a comfortable position.

Ask him if he wants anything before you leave.

Put the bell within his reach.

Leave the bed clean and neat.

Open the patient's screen or open the door.

Cover and remove the equipment.

Put any specimens into the right containers and label them.

Clean reusable equipment. Sterilize anything that requires it.

Throw disposables into the right container.

Wash your hands.

Mark down in the home chart: *the name of the treatment; the time of the treatment; the name of any medication or solution used and the amount; the condition of the patient before the treatment; the condition of the patient during the treatment; the condition of the patient after the treatment; a description of any drainage resulting from the treatment.*

2

Vital Signs

Temperature

Body temperature is the balance maintained between heat gener-
ated by the body and heat lost by the body.

Heat is made constantly by such body activities as digesting food,
making urine, breathing, circulating blood, walking, turning, and
lifting. Even thinking produces heat. The degree of heat made depends on the amount of activity and the blood supply to the active
area. The heart, kidneys, and liver are always active and have large
blood supplies, so they are hotter than other parts of the body. The
brain has a small supply of blood, and so, even with increased
activity, it is never very hot.

When infection occurs, and body resistance to disease increases,
body temperature rises.

The body loses heat constantly through skin exposure, the intake
of food and water, breathing, urinating, and other discharges.

So, in order to maintain a balance between heat made and heat
lost, the body must constantly regulate temperature. In health, this
regulation works so well that there are only slight changes in the
overall body temperature despite greatly increased activity. Illness
interferes with the body's ability to regulate its temperature; the
sicker the body, the greater the interference.

Taking the body temperature, then, is an excellent way to help
determine how ill the body is. And taking and recording the body
temperature at certain hours over a period of time is an excellent
way of determining the course of an illness.

Patients with fever and those in doubtful condition should have their temperatures taken every four hours in a twenty-four-hour period: 8:00 A.M., 12:00 noon, 4:00 P.M., 8:00 P.M., 12:00 midnight, and 4:00 A.M.

A patient who is not so ill might have his temperature taken less often. The 12 midnight and 4:00 A.M. temperatures may be omitted so that the patient may sleep without disturbance. Certain patients may need their temperatures taken only once or twice a day. The doctor may order how often to take a patient's temperature.

Temperature can be taken by using a thermometer in three ways: oral (by mouth); rectal (inserted into the anus); axillary (inside the armpit).

Oral Temperature

The mouth thermometer has a long slender silver tip. This tip is placed under the tongue and the lips are closed tightly around the thermometer. It is left in place for three minutes. The normal temperature by mouth is 98.6° F. (37° C.).

Rectal Temperature

The rectal thermometer has a fat bulblike silver tip. Lubricant is put on the tip and it is inserted into the anus (the opening of the rectum) for a distance of about three inches. It is left in place for three minutes. Normal rectal temperature is 99.6°F. (37.5° C.). A rectal temperature is always taken when there is any interference with the person's ability to breathe, when a patient is confused, and on a child. In the last two instances, the thermometer should always be inserted and held by you for the three minutes.

Axillary Temperature

Either an oral or rectal thermometer may be used to take an axillary temperature. The silver tip is placed well inside the armpit and the arm is held tight against the body. The thermometer is left in place for ten minutes. Normal axillary temperature is 97.6° F. (36° C.). An axillary temperature may be taken if neither an oral nor rectal temperature can be taken. EXAMPLE: On a baby with diarrhea.

Taking a Temperature

Equipment
    a pencil and paper or patient's home record
    a thermometer in a container of mouthwash solution
    a tissue
    a lubricant, if a rectal thermometer is used
    a wristwatch with a second hand

Remove the thermometer from its container of sterilizing solution.

Wipe it with a tissue.

Check the reading, shake, and recheck until the reading is below 96° F. (33° C.).

Insert the thermometer.

Note the time.

Count the pulse and respirations (see instructions on pages 24 and 25).

Record the pulse and respirations in the home record.

After three minutes (or ten for axillary) remove the thermometer.

Wipe it with a tissue, read (see below), and record the temperature in the home record.

Shake down the thermometer and return it to its container of mouthwash solution.

Reading a Thermometer

Have a good light.

Pinch the glass end of the thermometer with your thumb and first finger.

Raise the thermometer horizontally until it is level with your eyes.

Slowly roll the thermometer between your fingers until you see line markings along the top and numbers along the bottom. This is the correct reading position.

As you look between the line markings and the numbers, very

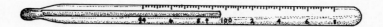

Reading a temperature on a rectal thermometer
(notice mercury at 99.6° F.)

slowly rotate the thermometer until you see a ribbon of silver or red. To read the temperature, look at the end of the ribbon, then at the nearest long mark. Read that number.

Then count 2 for each of the small markings going forward to the end of the ribbon. Read the last number and write both numbers like this: 99.6° F. (37.5° C.).

Thermometers

A small wad of cotton should be placed at the bottom of the thermometer container to prevent breaking or chipping the thermometer.

Never wash a thermometer in warm or hot water.

When shaking a thermometer, stand clear of nearby objects.

If a thermometer breaks in a patient's mouth: *tell the patient not to swallow; get him to spit out what he can; let him rinse his mouth and spit several times; examine his mouth for glass bits or cuts; report the accident to the doctor at once; in an emergency give bread if the patient has swallowed glass (bread collects the glass bits and lessens the chances of injury).*

The Pulse Rate

The pulse rate is the count of the heartbeat as it affects an artery. It is influenced by many things: a person's size, age, sex, posture, activity, emotions, and kind and degree of illness. A younger person has a faster normal pulse than a mature person. A female has a faster normal pulse than a male.

A normal pulse — that is, a pulse count taken when a person is resting — can be anywhere between 50 and 90.

Taking the Pulse

Place the tips of your three middle fingers along the inside of the patient's wrist just below his thumb. Roll your fingers over that area until you feel the pulse beat.

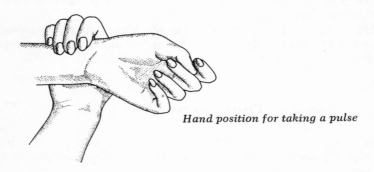

Hand position for taking a pulse

Use a watch with a second hand. Start counting the pulse beat when the second hand reaches 12. Count the beat for a full minute (until the second hand returns to 12).

Record the pulse count in the home record.

Respiration

Respiration is the process of breathing in and out. Since the process is continuous, only the breathing-in part of respiration, or inhalation, is counted to determine respiration rate.

The respiration count is affected by the same things that influence pulse count. In addition, the count is affected by the person's awareness that he is breathing or that his respirations are being counted. So it is important not to let the person know just when you count his respirations.

A normal respiration count — that is, a count taken when a person is resting — ranges from 16 to 24.

Counting Respirations

Place the patient's wrist so that it rests on his chest. Hold the wrist of the patient as though you were taking his pulse but release

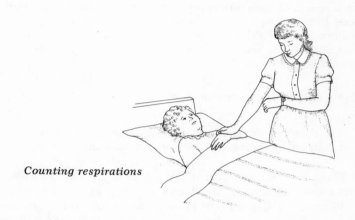

Counting respirations

the pressure of your fingers so as not to feel the pulse. Watch the patient's chest out of the corner of your eye.

Glance at the second hand of your watch. When that hand reaches 12, count as you feel each rise of the patient's chest. Count the rises for a full minute or until the second hand returns to 12.

Record the respiration in the home record.

Blood Pressure

Blood pressure is a method of measuring the force of blood against the walls of an artery, which depends on heart action and the elasticity of the artery. Blood pressure normally varies from one minute to the next, depending on a person's physical, mental, and emotional activity. An active person will have a higher pressure than a resting person.

Frequent blood pressure checks are important in the treatment of certain patients with heart or blood vessel diseases. In this situation, a doctor or a member of a health service will train a family member to take a patient's blood pressure. The patient should never take his own pressure, for the act of taking it changes the reading. Blood pressure should only be taken at the times indicated by the doctor, for example, every morning before breakfast and when and if the patient is excited. Sometimes three readings — done with the patient lying down, then sitting, then standing — are required at each specified time. Blood pressure can be taken on any limb of the body but is most often taken on the arm. Sometimes a doctor will require it to be taken on both arms or on all four limbs at each specified time. When only one arm is required, the same arm should always be used.

Using a Blood Pressure Machine

Equipment
  a stethoscope (a listening aid that magnifies sound)
  a sphygmomanometer (a blood pressure–measuring machine)

Place the patient's arm, palm up, in a natural position. Unless otherwise indicated by the doctor, either arm may be used.

Wrap the collapsed cuff around the upper arm above the elbow and place the arm so that the inner side of the elbow is exposed.

Be sure the cuff tube is attached to the dial tube.

Open the air lock on the bulb.

Find the patient's pulse just below the thumb of the same arm and keep your fingers on it.

Pump the bulb to fill the cuff with air. Fill until the pulse can no longer be felt. Filling the cuff forces the mercury or dial reading to act.

Lock the air inlet and release the pulse.

Place your stethoscope in position. Be sure the cone or disc sound lock is open. The earpieces go inside your ears. Press the cone or disc to the inner angle of the elbow below the cuff.

Watch the dial or meter.

Release the air lock as slowly as you can so that the mercury or dial slowly drops.

Take the following two readings:

Systolic. Listen for the first sound of a beat. Read the number on the dial or column when that sound is first heard.

Diastolic. Continue to listen until the last beat is heard. Read the number on the dial or column where the last beat is heard.

Release all air from the cuff.

Remove the cuff from the patient and write down the two readings in this manner.

B/P $\dfrac{120 \text{ the top reading is the systolic count}}{80 \text{ the lower reading is the diastolic count}}$

Record the blood pressure reading in the home chart.

3

Medicine

Government Control

Despite the control of medicine by federal law (the Pure Food and Drug Act), taking both prescription and nonprescription medicines in the United States is considered by most people to be necessary to everyday life. It is, in fact, so exaggerated that it is not at all uncommon to find people accustomed to taking several aspirins, several antacids, several tranquilizers, several diet pills, and a sleeping pill all in one day. Only in recent years has the American public begun to realize that it is being manipulated by the advertising of the drug companies into taking far more medicines than it needs. This manipulation results from our free enterprise system, which allows drugmaking and distributing to operate as competitive business opportunities. These businesses require advertising and drug buying on an ever-increasing scale in order to make money and to stay in business. The public, however, is suffering from this enterprise. Not only is it persuaded to take more medicines than it needs, but these unnecessary medicines are harmful to the body.

Although medicines can allay symptoms and sometimes cure disease, they can also produce undesirable and unexpected side effects, which vary with the individual. They can be mild, like a rash, headaches, depression, nausea, or drowsiness, or more severe, such as prolonged vomiting, bleeding, weakness, or changes in vision and hearing. Hence many medicines are prescription drugs; they are for the most part stronger and the danger of reaction therefore is greater. It is wrong to assume, however, that because a medicine is nonprescription it is safe and good to use. Medicine is not a natural need of the body. A good rule to follow is: Never take a medicine if relief of a symptom can be obtained by some other way. For example, taking a walk in the fresh air is a far better cure for an ordinary headache than an aspirin because a walk will often relieve the cause of the headache, while the pill relieves only the symptom.

When you do take nonprescription medicines, read all the information that is packaged with it. The law requires nonprescription medicines to list warnings about possible side effects. If an undesired reaction occurs, stop taking the medicine at once. If the reaction is strong consult a doctor or an emergency service at once.

Prescriptions

When a doctor gives you a prescription, get him to tell you as much as possible about it. You have the right to the following information:

the name of the medicine and the strength ordered
why it is being given to you
what beneficial effects to expect from it
what possible side effects to watch for
how much of the medicine you are to take at each dose
how often to take a dose; whether timing should be exact or as needed
if the medicine might react with any other medicine that you are presently taking
the best time to take the medicine (before meals, after meals, etc.)
if there is any reason not to skip a dose or to discontinue taking the medicine before the prescription runs out
if the prescription can be refilled

Ask the doctor to write this information on a piece of paper for you.

Never take a medicine if you do not know these things. If you have ever had a bad reaction to a medicine, be sure and tell the doctor *each time he gives you a prescription*. You cannot rely on him always to remember that you react unfavorably to medicine.

When you take your prescription to be filled, check the label on the medicine that you receive.

A pharmacist, a person licensed by state law to prepare and dispense medicines, fills a doctor's prescription.

Any prescription is always labeled. The label tells the following very important facts:

the patient's name
the prescription order number
the doctor's name
how the medicine is to be given (EXAMPLE: by mouth)
when the medicine is to be given (EXAMPLE: every four hours except when sleeping)
how much of the medicine is to be given at any one time (EXAMPLE: two tablets for first dose, one tablet thereafter)
whether the medicine needs special care (EXAMPLE: refrigerate)

Be sure that the information on the label matches the information given to you by the doctor. If it doesn't, ask the pharmacist why it is different and to check the prescription. If there is a difference between what the doctor has written and the information he has given you, have the pharmacist call the doctor. If the pharmacist has made a mistake, do not accept the medicine. Take your prescription to another pharmacy.

Never take or give to anyone medicine that has been prescribed for someone else. Do not keep prescription medicines beyond the time for which they are ordered. Some medicines deteriorate and can cause undesirable effects if taken. Some medicines must be taken in regulated quantity and spacing or the results can be harmful. Leftover medicines tempt one to take them unnecessarily. Get rid of them.

Some Common Medicines

Nonprescription, or Over-the-Counter

ANTACIDS (Tums, Rolaids, etc.)
Chew tablet antacids thoroughly before swallowing. Follow with a glass of water.

Shake liquid antacids thoroughly before taking. Follow with a glass of water or milk.

Constipation may result from taking certain antacids over a period of several days.

Some antacids contain sugar and should not be used by diabetics.

Antacids should not be used together with certain other medicines. Be sure and tell your doctor that you take antacids before he writes a prescription for you.

Baking soda should not be taken frequently or without a doctor's knowledge.

ASPIRIN, PAIN RELIEVERS

Aspirin is found in many nonprescription medicines that relieve pain: Alka-Seltzer, Anacin, Aspergum, Bufferin, Cope, Edrisal, Empirin Compound, Midol, Excedrin, etc. Therefore the same rules that apply to aspirin apply to all.

To prevent decomposition, aspirin should be kept in a tight container. Exposed aspirins should be discarded.

The container should be stored out of the reach of children. Aspirin overdose is the major cause of poisoning in children. (Some manufacturers package aspirin products in containers with special lids that are difficult for children to open.)

Aspirin can irritate the stomach lining. It should always be taken after meals or with milk.

If taken thirty minutes before planned exercise or physical therapy by a person with painful joints, the pain relief will allow freer movement.

Aspirin increases perspiration, so care should be taken to prevent exposure to chill.

BOWEL STIMULANTS

Cathartics (castor oil, Cascara Sagrada, Ducolax, milk of magnesia, Epsom salts, mineral oil). Frequent use of strong cathartics is discouraged by most doctors.

Coated tablets should never be chewed, but swallowed whole.

Shake milk of magnesia before taking. Follow with water or fruit juice to increase effectiveness.

Take castor oil, Epsom salts, and Ducolax before breakfast. Milk of magnesia, Cascara Sagrada, and mineral oil may be taken at bedtime.

The taste of castor oil, Epsom salts, or mineral oil may be removed from the mouth if the patient sucks on a wedge of orange after taking the medicine.

Straining during bowel movements should be avoided. It interferes with normal heart and blood vessel action.

Frequent use of mineral oil prevents the body from absorbing certain vitamins from the intestines.

Laxatives (Hydrolose, Mucelose, Serutan). Effective and gentle-working cellulose that swells the intestine, softens stools, and stimulates intestinal movement. Swallow whole and follow with one or two glasses of water.

COLD OR "ALLERGY" MEDICINE

Most cold and allergy medicines, whether liquid, pills, or capsules, contain antihistamine, and the same rules for antihistamines should be followed when taking these medicines.

Many cold and allergy pills contain aspirin, and the same rules for taking aspirin should be followed when taking these medicines.

DIET PILLS

Most diet pills contain ingredients that draw water from body cells and increase urination. Use for extended periods of time or without the knowledge of your doctor can lead to changes in blood chemistry and symptoms such as drowsiness, confusion, nausea, air hunger, a rash, and double vision.

Some diet pills contain ingredients that stimulate the central nervous system to decrease fatigue and produce feelings of well-being. Extended use may cause nervousness, dizziness, anxiety, confusion, headache, nausea, sweating, dry mouth and nose, and depression.

Some diet pills contain certain ingredients that swell in the intestine and act as a laxative. These should be swallowed with one or two glasses of water.

MENSTRUAL OR PREMENSTRUAL PILLS

These medicines may contain some of the same ingredients as diet pills and the same care should be used when taking them as when taking diet pills. In addition, they often contain aspirin, so the same care should be used as when taking aspirin.

VITAMINS AND MINERALS

Federal food and drug laws have restricted the amounts of Vitamins A and D available to the public without a prescription. Overdosage of these vitamins can cause toxic buildup in the body with resulting undesirable damage.

Caution should be used in taking B vitamins. B vitamins require balancing; too much of one can create a body deficiency in one or more of the other B vitamins.

Recent medical research indicates that large daily dosages of Vitamin C are not harmful to the body and do improve resistance to certain viral diseases.

Vitamins should be taken after rather than before a meal. Concentrated vitamins taken on an empty stomach can cause nausea and/or vomiting.

Iron tablets or a multivitamin — a mineral capsule containing iron — causes the stool to turn black in color. Iron can cause changes in bowel regularity, such as constipation or diarrhea.

Antacids and milk interfere with body absorption of iron and should not be taken together with any product containing iron.

DIARRHEA MEDICINE (Intestinal cramps) (Donnagel, Kaopectate, etc.)

Shake well before use.

Do not give to children under six years of age. Ask the doctor about treating diarrhea in young children.

Do not give more than four doses in one twenty-four-hour period.

Do not use if patient has a high fever.

Stop using if blurred vision, dizziness, or rapid pulse occurs.

Prescription

ANTIBIOTICS AND ANTIBACTERIALS

Given to increase resistance to certain infectious organisms.

It is important to take all of the total number of doses ordered by the doctor and to take each dose at the exact time indicated. Never skip a dose or discontinue without the doctor's knowledge. This can lower the strength of the medical offense against the disease organism and in some cases cause the organism to develop a resistance to the medicine, thereby reducing its effectiveness.

These drugs work best on an empty stomach and should be taken half an hour before or two hours after a meal.

Antacids reduce the effectiveness of these medicines and should not be taken with them.

Some of these medicines destroy intestinal bacteria that control the growth of another intestinal organism. Uncontrolled, this latter organism can spread to other areas of the body such as the mouth or vagina where it can cause inflammation and itching. Careful mouth care several times daily and washing the anal, or rectal, area after each bowel movement helps control the organism. If symptoms do develop, notify the doctor, who can order other medicine to check the growth of this organism.

Some of these medicines are very effective against specific organisms but ineffective against others. The doctor chooses the right medicine for each infection. If the doctor is unsure about which medicine to use, he will take a sample of the organism to determine its nature by culture and microscopic examination. Because the choice of medicine is so important, it is equally important not to use leftover antibiotics or antibacterials for another infection or for another person without the doctor's consent.

Some antibiotics decompose with age and can then be toxic to the body. When a prescription for antibiotics is discontinued, do not save the leftover medicine to use at another time.

Some people have allergic reactions to certain antibiotics. Any unusual symptoms such as a rash, itching, vomiting, or diarrhea should be reported to the doctor at once.

When taking antibiotics or antibacterials, fluid intake should be increased.

ANTIHISTAMINES

These medicines block the action of histamine and produce a sedative effect. They are given to relieve symptoms of such problems as asthma, hay fever, allergic rashes, and serum reactions.

Because drowsiness and/or blurred vision often occurs after taking an antihistamine, a consumer should not drive or do industrial work.

Care should be taken ascending or descending stairs.

The consumer should smoke only when another person is present.

Undesirable effects such as headache, nausea, dry mouth, nervousness, irritability, or excitement should be reported to the doctor.

PAIN RELIEVERS (Narcotics)

Some narcotics may cause constipation.

Dizziness and drowsiness are common.

A patient should not drive or do other work requiring mental alertness, judgment, and physical concentration.

Habitual use may cause addiction.

The patient should never smoke while alone.

Some people have reverse effects from certain narcotics (they may become excited, restless, etc.).

Use nursing measures such as a relaxing bath to help relieve pain and enhance the effects of the narcotic. SEE: Pain.

TRANQUILIZERS (Antianxiety medicines)

A patient should be very frank with his doctor about all previous physical or mental disorders since certain conditions do not favor the use of certain tranquilizers.

Use during pregnancy should be avoided.

Use while drinking alcohol should be avoided.

A patient should not drive or do other work requiring mental alertness, judgment, and physical coordination.

Take after meals.

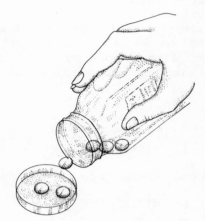

Measure tablets by pouring them into the bottle cap.

Sometimes causes appetite increase with resulting weight gain. Can cause mouth dryness and drowsiness.

Prolonged usage can lead to dependence.

General Rules for Giving Medicines

Before giving a medicine, check to see that you know

    the correct person;
    the correct medicine;
    the correct amount;
    the correct time;
    the correct way to give it.

Make out a twenty-four-hour medicine time sheet that lists all the patient's medicines and the times they are to be given. Next to each, write the amount and how it is to be given. Then you need only look at the sheet to know which amount of what medication your patient should take at what hour.

EXAMPLE: The patient has five different medicines. Check your watch with the medicine time sheet. Check the prescription number, the amount, and directions on the time sheet.

Read the complete label before opening any medicine bottle. Check the label against the time sheet information.

Pour the medicine. If it is in tablet or capsule form, shake the correct number to be given into the cap of the bottle and then use the cap to pour that number into a small, dry glass.

Read the label again before you close the medicine bottle.

Check all the information about the poured medicine again.

Close the bottle and return it to safe storage.

TIME	PRESCRIPTION NUMBER	AMOUNT	DIRECTIONS
6:00 A.M.	#18932	1 cap.	one capsule by mouth every four hours night and day
7:30 A.M.	#26705	2 tab.	two tablets by mouth before meals three times a day
10:00 A.M.	#18932	1 cap.	as at 6:00 A.M.
10:00 A.M.	#37602	1 tab.	1 tablet by mouth every day
10:00 A.M.	#43102	1 t.	one teaspoon by mouth every morning
11:30 A.M.	#26705	2 tab.	as at 7:30 A.M.
2:00 P.M.	#18932	1 cap.	as at 6:00 A.M.
5:30 P.M.	#26705	2 tab.	as at 7:30 A.M.
6:00 P.M.	#18932	1 cap.	as at 6:00 A.M.
10:00 P.M.	#18932	1 cap.	as at 6:00 A.M.
10:00 P.M.	#23401	1 suppository	(rectal) at bedtime (refrigerate)
2:00 A.M.	#18932	1 cap.	as at 6:00 A.M.

Give the medicine to the patient.

Stay with the patient until the medicine is taken.

Watch for and report any unusual symptom that might be a reaction to the medicine.

Write down when the medicine was given and how the patient accepted it. Do this at once, so that there is no possibility of an extra dose being given.

Taking Medicines

Most patients take several kinds of medicine each day. Whenever possible, doctors prefer patients to be in charge of taking their own medications. Self-medication is therefore allowed in many home-care, day-care, and minimal-care nursing home situations. The following methods help to remind the patient to take his medicine and to check on whether he has done so.

Have separate containers for each kind of medicine but give the patient the amounts he will use on a daily basis. EXAMPLE: If his prescription calls for one capsule three times a day, each morning give him a container with three capsules.

See that each container is correctly marked with prescription information.

Make out a daily twenty-four-hour medicine time sheet for the patient to refer to. Go over the sheet with him to be sure that he understands it. Each time he takes a medicine, he can cross it off the list.

If he must take medicine at a set hour, give him an alarm clock with the alarm set for the correct time.

See that he has access to whatever he may need to take with the medicine, such as water or milk.

Giving Medicines at Home

Unless a medicine needs special care, all of the patient's medicine bottles should be kept together, apart from medicines belonging to other family members. All medicines should be out of reach of children or animals.

By Mouth

Equipment
    a glass of fresh water
    a small glass or paper cup for the medicine

a measure (if needed)
a slice of fruit or a cracker (if the medicine tastes bad)

Some medicines must be given with food. This is indicated on the label. If taken at a time other than mealtime, a glass of milk is usually given.

To the Skin

Equipment
a setup for whatever the treatment requires: soaks, compresses, and so forth

By Injection

No one should give an injection except in unusual circumstances and under the instruction and supervision of a doctor or professional nurse. SEE: Diabetes.

Equipment
sterile syringes and needles of the right size (usually disposable), available by prescription
a sterile alcohol wiper for preparing the skin

Through Inhalation

SEE: Heart and Lung Disease.

By Rectal Suppository

Rectal suppositories, always ordered by the doctor, are small cones of glycerine, cocoa butter, soap, or other such easily melted substance. A cone is put through the anus and into the rectum.

Cones may be plain or medicated. Because they melt easily, they are always kept in the refrigerator.

Often one is given to stimulate bowel function or soften a hard mass of feces. Sometimes one is given to be retained and its medicine quickly absorbed into the bloodstream by the many blood vessels around the anus. SEE: Toileting (Enemas).

Equipment
the suppository
a disposable plastic glove or finger cot
a lubricant

Follow the general rules for treatments.

Place the patient in the position for giving an enema in bed. SEE: Enemas.

Put on the glove.

Lubricate the first or index finger.

Use the finger to massage the anus and relax it.

Take the suppository between the thumb and index finger of the gloved hand.

Separate the buttocks with the other hand.

Insert the suppository gently into the anus.

Push it well past the anus by inserting the tip of your index finger. If the anus is lax, press a sanitary napkin against it and hold for at least ten minutes.

4

Sleep, Rest, and Physical Therapy

Sleep

In recent years studies have been made of sleep and brain activity during sleep. Researchers have found that in the process of sleeping, the brain goes through several distinct changes in activity. One of these changes is called REM (Rapid Eye Movement), because the eyes jerk restlessly beneath closed lids.

REM sleep is associated with dreaming. Studies show that dreaming is essential for health. Deprived of dream sleep, any person becomes irritable, loses muscle control, and grows mentally confused. During the next dream sleep period, a person will dream more often to make up for lost dreaming time. All people, therefore, need sufficient dream sleep.

Older people, however, do not seem to require the average eight hours of continuous sleep needed by most younger adults. Older patients may sleep only a few continuous hours, awakening often to urinate, to drink water, to eat snacks, to listen to the radio, to read, and the like. Sometimes they seem to awaken only to reassure themselves that they are in familiar surroundings.

Although each person's sleeping pattern differs, most have preparatory rituals for sleep.

People can be very specific in their wants and in the exact placement of things. One might want the shade of a lamp positioned just so, a bedpan or urinal placed on a chair within easy reach, a radio on a special corner of the bedside table, eyeglasses and tissues positioned on the table, an extra pillow, or a certain blanket.

Sometimes the demands can seem time-consuming and unnecessary, but the patient will respond very well to your tolerance in meeting his demands. He will feel secure and will sleep better.

Rest

Besides night sleep, many patients require several rest and nap periods during the day. Most doctors recommend an hour or two of rest after the midday meal, when the patient may want to go to bed. Other rest periods should be arranged to suit the patient's need. Many older patients are able to doze while sitting, even in crowded or noisy situations.

When a patient is expected to walk an unusual distance or climb many stairs, a small lightweight chair can be taken along. Then he can stop to rest whenever he feels the need.

Insomnia

Insomnia is the inability to sleep. It may be temporary and related to immediate stress or long-term and related to individual biochemical rhythms.

Signs of insomnia are yawning; irritability; nervousness; over-tiredness; reddened, puffy, or drooping eyelids; dark skin under the eyes; dizziness; lack of coordination; mental confusion; muscular tension.

Provide a calm, serene, comfortable sleeping situation for the patient.

Allow the patient to do whatever he is accustomed to do at bedtime: take a bath, read, listen to music.

Use other relaxing comfort measures, such as deep breathing exercises, a hot water bottle at the feet, a massage, an alcohol sponge bath, or a glass of milk.

Physical Therapy

Physical therapy is treatment through stimulation of the body or a body part. The aims of physical therapy are

to maintain and increase normal body function;
to prevent loss of function when possible;

to train a patient to substitute functioning when loss occurs; to help a patient become as independent as possible.

Specific physical therapy for the individual patient is ordered by the doctor after testing and evaluation. A patient's program may include more than one of the following:

range of motion exercises
activities of daily living
use of special equipment, such as Hubbard tank, Whirlpool
    bath, ultrasound, or a hot wax bath
occupational therapy
recreational therapy

Body Joints

The normal extent of motion in a human depends on the ways in which his 206 bones are joined to form the body skeleton. When one bone connects to another so that a part of the body is movable, the bone connection is called a joint.

Here are some main kinds of joints.

CONDYLOID JOINT
Two bones connect to allow angle movement in two directions. EXAMPLE: wrists.

BALL-AND-SOCKET JOINT
Two bones connect to allow movement in all directions. EXAMPLES: shoulders and hips.

GLIDING JOINT
Two bones connect by sliding against each other. EXAMPLES: small bones of the wrists and ankles.

HINGE JOINT
Two bones connect to allow angle movement in one direction. EXAMPLES: elbows and knees.

PIVOT JOINT
Two bones connect to allow one to rotate around part of the other. EXAMPLES: spinal bones.

Body Motion

Activity or body motion is important to the health of any individual of any age. Motion increases blood circulation, which improves the functioning of all body parts, in particular the cardiovascular and respiratory systems. Motion also

helps maintain the range of movement in body joints;
prevents deformities by keeping joints moving freely;
increases the range of joint movement in people with decreased range of movement;
helps maintain muscle strength;
increases muscle strength after loss of strength following sickness or injury;
helps maintain good coordination of the nervous system;
aids all healing, helps prevent swelling of the legs and feet, and helps prevent skin breakdown;
increases a person's endurance (the ability to perform the same movement over and over during a length of time).

A younger person makes enough natural motions in his daily routine to keep his body functioning. He also seeks exercise, such as swimming, playing tennis, and dancing.

Aging causes a gradual slowing of all body activities. Unless a plan of activity is carried out, an older person loses more and more of his ability to perform full motions. A plan of activity can mean the difference between a patient becoming a helpless invalid and being able to care for himself.

The plan of activity is ordered by the doctor to suit the patient's individual need. It may vary from a daily walk to special exercises for different parts of the patient's body.

Special exercises needed by the patient are determined by testing the extent of movement in his joints and the extent of self-care he can perform. These special exercises are called range of motion exercises.

Range of Motion (ROM)

Range of motion means the full extent of movement in a body joint.

Normal range of motion means the ability to perform a full movement of a body joint.

Functional range of motion means a less than normal ability to move a body joint but enough ability to allow a person to perform activities of daily living.

Activities of daily living (ADL) are movements made in the course of daily self-care. An ROM test is used to determine the extent of ROM in a patient. Based on the results of this test, a doctor can prescribe specific exercises to suit the patient's needs. The patient is retested regularly and his exercise program adjusted accordingly.

ROM EXERCISES

Free active ROM exercises are done entirely by the patient.

Resistive ROM exercises are done by a patient against pull provided by another person, a weight, or a machine.

Active assistance ROM exercises are done in part by the patient and in part by another person or a machine.

Passive ROM exercises are done to a patient by another person or machine without any help from the patient.

A prescription for ROM exercises on a particular patient may require the use of one or more kinds of motion exercises. EXAMPLE: A patient may need free active ROM exercises for his shoulders, resistive ROM exercises for one arm, and passive ROM exercises for both legs.

USING ROM EXERCISES

ROM exercises are most effective when done at regular, frequent intervals, and when one motion is repeated a limited number of times. For example, it is better to do an ROM exercise twice a day for five times at each exercise period than once a day for ten times.

BEFORE ROM EXERCISES

Dress the patient so that he can move freely and without embarrassment.

Get the full attention and cooperation of the patient.

Put the patient at ease.

Before each new exercise, describe it to the patient. Tell him in what ways it should affect and help him. Tell the patient how he should feel while the exercise is being done.

Tell him what he should do during the exercise.

If the exercise is *free active,* tell the patient to perform it alone.

If the exercise is *resistive,* tell the patient to pull against the resistance.

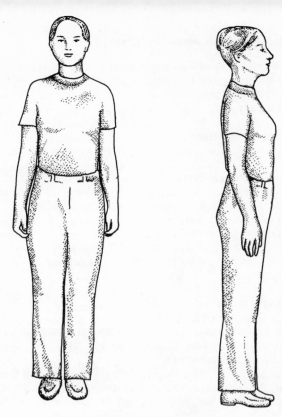

NEUTRAL POSITION — STANDING

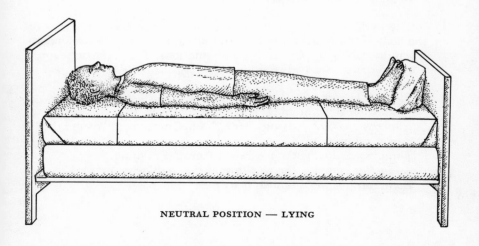

NEUTRAL POSITION — LYING

If the exercise is *active assistive*, explain to the patient how he should help during the movement.

If the exercise is *passive*, tell the patient to relax the body part and keep it limp.

DURING ROM EXERCISES

Inspire the patient with confidence in your ability to exercise him.

Encourage his self-confidence.

Make sure that all movements are as complete as possible.

Make sure that all movements are smooth and steady.

Do not overtire the patient.

Do not cause unnecessary pain.

Be alert for unfavorable changes in the patient, such as pain or unusual weakness or pallor. Stop the exercise session if any of these occurs.

AFTER ROM EXERCISES

See that the patient is comfortable.

Record in the home record any changes noticed in the patient either between the last exercise period and the present one or changes during the treatment.

Neutral Position. Standing or lying straight with heels together and arms at the sides and palms toward the body is called the neutral position. This position can be assumed in the following lying positions:

Lateral: lying on one side
Prone: lying on the abdomen and face
Supine: lying on the back

The midline is an imaginary line dividing the body or a part of the body lengthwise into two equal halves. It is used as a reference when describing or performing body motions. The following words are used to describe body motions:

Flexion: bending
Extension: straightening
Hyperextension: carrying a straightened movement beyond the neutral position
Abduction: moving the part away from the midline
Adduction: moving the part toward the midline
Rotation: turning a limb or body part

1. Start with head in neutral position.

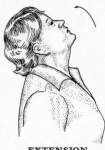

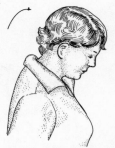

EXTENSION
looking up

FLEXION
looking down

2. Start with head in neutral position.

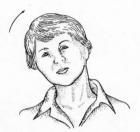

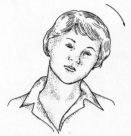

RIGHT LATERAL FLEXION
*bending head toward
right shoulder*

LEFT LATERAL FLEXION
*bending head toward
left shoulder*

3. Start with head in neutral position.

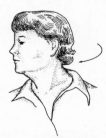

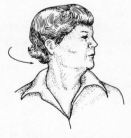

RIGHT ROTATION
*turning head to right
to see over shoulder*

LEFT ROTATION
*turning head to left
to see over shoulder*

* **FOR PASSIVE ROM:** Cup your hands over the patient's ears and grasp the head
in a firm hold.

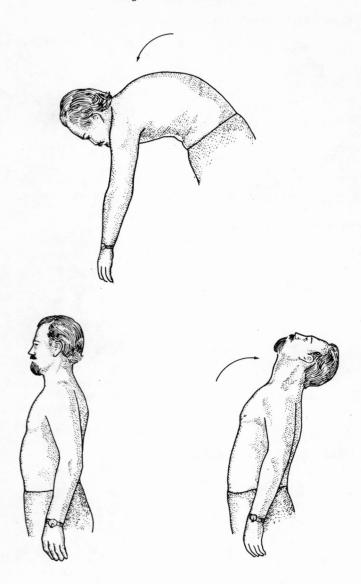

1. Start with body in neutral position.

* FOR PASSIVE ROM: Reach around the patient's back to grasp his far shoulder with one of your hands, allowing the patient's head to rest on your forearm. Grasp the patient's near shoulder with your other hand. As an alternative, hold both of the patient's legs at the knees with one or both hands, while the patient rotates his trunk.

2. Start with body in neutral position.

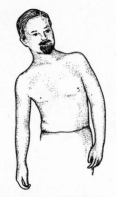 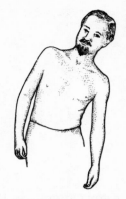

RIGHT LATERAL FLEXION
bending sideways to right

LEFT LATERAL FLEXION
bending sideways to left

3. Start with body in neutral position.

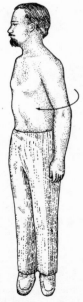 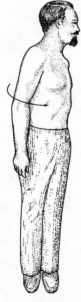

RIGHT ROTATION
turning shoulders to right

LEFT ROTATION
turning shoulders to left

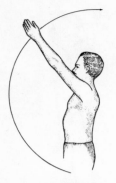 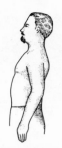 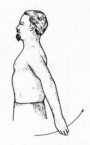

FLEXION
*moving arm forward
and upward*

EXTENSION
*returning arm
to neutral position*

HYPEREXTENSION
*moving arm backward
from neutral position*

1. Start with arm in neutral postion.*

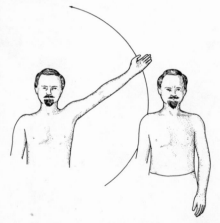

VERTICAL ABDUCTION
*moving arm sideways,
away from the body and
over the head*

VERTICAL ADDUCTION
*returning arm to neutral
position*

2. Start with arm in neutral position.†

* FOR PASSIVE ROM: Stand facing the side of the patient to be exercised. Place your near hand just above the patient's elbow. Use your other hand to support the patient's wrist and hand.
† FOR PASSIVE ROM: Stand facing the front or back of the patient. Grasp the patient's arm just above the elbow. Use your other hand to support the patient's wrist and hand.

3. Start with arm at shoulder height and elbow bent at a right angle.*

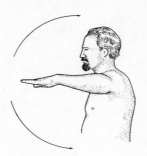

EXTERNAL ROTATION
turning the upper part of the arm so that the forearm and palm face forward

INTERNAL ROTATION
turning the upper part of the arm so that the forearm and palm face backward

4. Start with arm at shoulder height and elbow straight.†

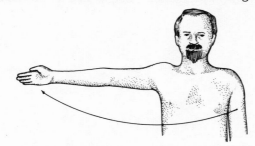

HORIZONTAL ABDUCTION
moving arm back as far as possible

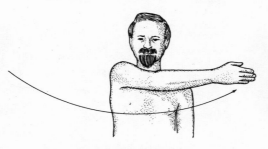

HORIZONTAL ADDUCTION
moving arm forward across the chest

* FOR PASSIVE ROM: With the patient on his back, face the arm to be exercised. With one hand, grasp the patient's arm just below the elbow. Use your other hand to support the patient's wrist and hand.
† FOR PASSIVE ROM: Stand facing patient's head on side to be exercised. Grasp the patient's arm just above the elbow. Use your other hand to support the patient's hand and wrist.

5. Start with arm in neutral position.*

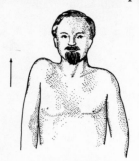 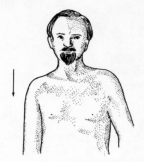

ELEVATION
lifting shoulder

DEPRESSION
lowering shoulder

6. Start with arm at shoulder height in forward flexion.†

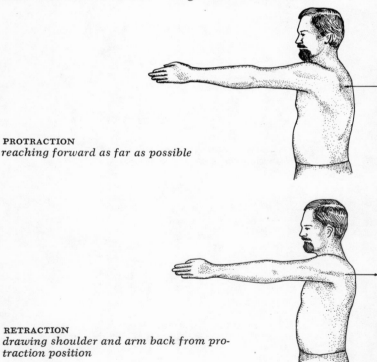

PROTRACTION
reaching forward as far as possible

RETRACTION
*drawing shoulder and arm back from pro-
traction position*

---

* FOR PASSIVE ROM: Stand facing patient's head on side to be exercised. Grasp the patient's arm just above the elbow. Use your other hand to support the patient's hand and wrist.
† FOR PASSIVE ROM: Stand facing patient's side to be exercised. Grasp the patient's arm just above the elbow. Use your other hand to support the patient's hand and wrist.

Start with arm in neutral position.

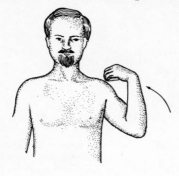 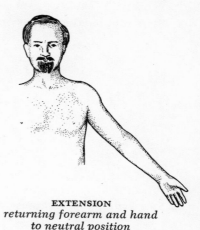

FLEXION
bending elbow and bringing fore-
arm and hand toward shoulder

EXTENSION
returning forearm and hand
to neutral position

Elbow Motions*

Start with elbow at waist, bent at a right angle, with palm facing
body.

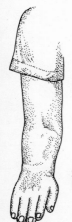 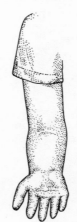

PRONATION
turning palm downward

SUPLINATION
turning palm upward

Forearm Motions†

* FOR PASSIVE ROM: Stand facing the arm to be exercised. Grasp the patient's arm
just above the elbow. Use your other hand to support the patient's wrist and hand.
† FOR PASSIVE ROM: Use both your hands to grasp the patient's hand and wrist.

Wrist Motions*

1. Start with hand in extension.

   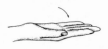

FLEXION
*bending wrist so that
palm faces forearm*

EXTENSION
*returning hand
to starting position*

HYPEREXTENSION
*moving hand so that
the back of it faces
the forearm*

2. Start with hand in extension.

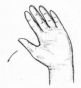

RADICAL DEVIATION
*moving hand
sideways so that
thumb is toward
forearm*

ULNAR DEVIATION
*moving hand side-
ways so that little
finger is toward
forearm*

Finger Motions

1. Start with hand in extension.†

FLEXION
making a fist

EXTENSION
opening hand

2. Start with hand in extension.‡

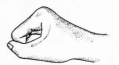

ABDUCTION
spreading fingers

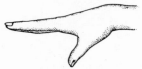

ADDUCTION
closing fingers

---

* FOR PASSIVE ROM: Use one of your hands to grasp the patient's arm just above
the wrist. Use your other hand to hold the patient's hand.

† FOR PASSIVE ROM: Use one of your hands to support the patient's forearm and
wrist. Use the fingers of your other hand to open and close the patient's fingers.

‡ FOR PASSIVE ROM: Use both of your hands to hold the fingers of one of the patient's hands.

Thumb Motions*

1. Start with thumb in extension.

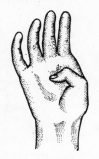
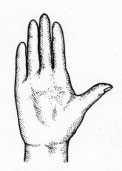

FLEXION
bending all joints

EXTENSION
straightening all joints

2. Start with hand, palm upward, in extension.

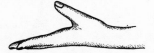
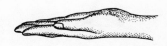

ABDUCTION
raising thumb

ADDUCTION
returning thumb

3. Start with hand in extension.

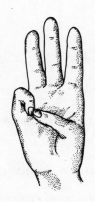

OPPOSITION
*touching tips of thumb and
little finger*

* FOR PASSIVE ROM: Support the patient's hand and fingers with one of your
hands. Use your other hand to hold the patient's thumb.

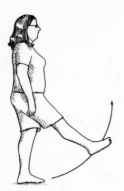 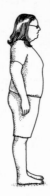 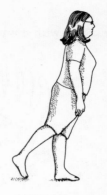

FLEXION
*moving leg for-
ward from hip*

EXTENSION
*returning leg to
neutral position*

HYPEREXTENSION
*moving leg back
from hip*

1. Start with leg in neutral position.*

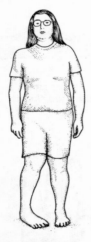 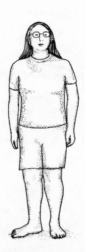

INTERNAL ROTATION
turning leg and toes inward

EXTERNAL ROTATION
turning leg and toes outward

2. Start with leg in neutral position.†

* **FOR PASSIVE ROM:** *Flexion and Extension.* Support the patient's leg by placing his ankle on your arm or shoulder. Place your hand over his knee to keep it straight. *Hyperextension.* Turn patient onto his abdomen. Place one of your hands under the patient's ankle and grasp it. Place your other hand just above his knee.

† **FOR PASSIVE ROM:** Stand facing side to be exercised. Grasp the patient's ankle with one hand. Place your other hand on top of the knee.

3. Start with leg in neutral position.*

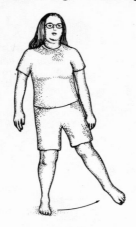

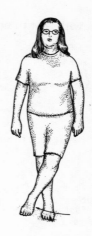

ABDUCTION
moving one leg outward

ADDUCTION
*returning leg to neutral position
and crossing it over the other leg*

Knee Motions†

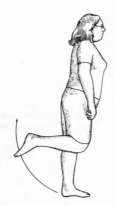

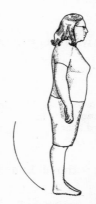

FLEXION
*bending knee and moving foot
toward back of leg*

EXTENSION
*returning leg
to neutral position*

Start with leg in neutral position.

* FOR PASSIVE ROM: Stand facing the side to be exercised. Place one hand just above the knee. Use your other hand to support the ankle.
† FOR PASSIVE ROM: With the patient on his back, put his hip in flexion and bend the knee. Support the leg by placing one of your hands just above the knee. Use your other hand to grasp the ankle from beneath. As an alternative, turn the patient onto his abdomen, place one hand on the back of the leg just above the knee and use the other hand to grasp the ankle from beneath.

Ankle Motions

1. Start with foot in neutral position.*

DORSAL FLEXION
*moving foot and
toes toward the
shin*

PLANTAR FLEXION
*moving foot and
toes toward
the heel*

2. Start with foot in neutral position.†

EVERSION
*turning foot and
toes outward*

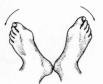
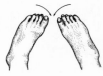

INVERSION
*turning foot and
toes inward*

Toe Motions

1. Start with foot in neutral position.‡

FLEXION
*bending toes
toward sole*

EXTENSION
*bending toes
toward shin*

2. Start with foot in neutral position.§

ABDUCTION
spreading toes

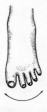

ADDUCTION
*returning toes to
neutral position*

* FOR PASSIVE ROM: Place one hand on the patient's knee to prevent flexion. With your other hand, hold the patient's foot so that the heel rests in your palm and the sole rests against your forearm.
† FOR PASSIVE ROM: Use one hand to hold the patient's heel. With the other hand, grasp the top of the foot.
‡ FOR PASSIVE ROM: Hold patient's foot with one hand. Use your other hand to move the toes.
§ FOR PASSIVE ROM: Use both hands to grasp the patient's toes.

Activities of Daily Living (ADL)

Activities of daily living are motions of self-care that are learned by the child and become habit with the adult. They include:

moving about in bed
personal grooming
dressing and undressing
eating
using one's hands
walking
using the toilet

Many health conditions can affect a patient's ability to do these things.

A patient is given regular ADL tests to determine his limitations and changes in his abilities to perform self-care. After each test, a specific ADL program is designed for the patient who needs reminding, remotivating, or retraining to help him perform these activities to the best of his ability. Such a program cannot succeed unless everyone concerned works with the patient and with the ADL instructor. A patient is usually hospitalized during his intensive instruction. Then family members are instructed in helping him with a specific program before he is allowed to go home. Both patient and family members may return for additional instruction if needed.

Caring for a patient on an ADL program requires understanding that

good balance is needed to perform independent self-care;
any self-care activity is made up of many steps, and sometimes a patient must conquer these steps one by one;
the patient constantly needs your patience and encouragement.

You can best help your patient with ADL activities by doing the following things:

Use the same words every day to instruct and encourage the patient. Make these words clear, simple, and brief.

Don't rush the patient. Allow him time to complete an activity at his own pace.

Find out if the patient is more interested in one activity than in another. Concentrate on the activity that interests him until he masters it.

See that the patient gets ADL training at the time when he would normally perform that activity. EXAMPLE: If an incontinent patient usually has a bowel movement each morning after breakfast, bowel retraining should be done at that time.

Allow the patient to do as much for himself as he is able.

Help him to master and use any adaptive equipment that may have been ordered for him.

See that adaptive equipment is in good working order and ready for the patient's use.

Position adaptive equipment so that the patient has easy access to it or can best use it.

Here are some of the many adaptive devices used in ADL. Most are available at local drugstores or medical supply houses. Often the patient, members of his family, and the ADL instructor work together to devise ingenious things that suit the patient's particular needs.

MOVING ABOUT IN BED
rope pull
trapeze

PERSONAL GROOMING
nail clipper
suction cup nailbrush
soap on a cord (to wear around the neck)
bath mitt
reachers to hold washcloth, powder puff, and other objects
curlers of self-fastening material, such as Velcro
long-handled bath brush or sponge
bathtub seat with back rest
wheelchair with commode seat for incontinent patient
spray deodorant
built-up handles on water faucets

DRESSING AND UNDRESSING
long-handled clothing hook
loops sewed on clothing to use with clothing hook

larger-sized clothing of stretch materials
clothing with front openings
trousers with elastic tops
Velcro self-closing fasteners
large buttons
a device for putting on stockings
elastic shoelaces
long-handled shoehorn
elastic cuff links

EATING

utensils with built-up handles
utensils with long handles
utensils with rockers
utensils with swivels
ADL palm cuff to hold various utensils
drinking straws
unbreakable dishes and glassware
spillproof edges on dishes and glassware
suction mat under dish to prevent slipping

USING THE HANDS

book rest
page turner
special telephone arms
weighted pencils, checkers, and other objects
clip clothespin with peg (for holding pencil or pen)
embroidery hoop with table clamp
rubber doorknob lever
car door opener
easy-open coin purse
holder for knitting, crocheting, and other needlecrafts
playing card holder
card shuffler
left-handed scissors

MOBILITY

braces
canes
crutches
walkers
wheelchairs

USING THE TOILET
    long-handled tongs for self-wiping
    grab bars for toilet
    built-up toilet seat

Remember that, in working with your patient in his ADL program, the best and fastest way for you to work can only be the best and fastest way possible for him.

Occupational Therapy

Occupational therapy can also provide physical therapy. It aims

    to occupy the mind and interest of a patient;
    to increase a patient's activity;
    to develop specific control of physical abilities;
    to train a patient for a job.

Therapy such as tooling leather or weaving is given to a patient to increase range of motion, strength, coordination, and agility in a specific body part that needs such building.

Recreational Therapy

The care of any patient, except one in critical condition, should include a plan for relaxing recreation adapted to his specific needs and interests.

The word "recreation" means to begin anew. In practice, recreation does more than that. It turns the mind away from pressures and worries and toward satisfactions. It relaxes the mind and so relaxes the body, which is an important part of health. Recreation is important as a stimulant to recovery from an illness or adjustment to illness.

There are two kinds of recreation, things that can be done alone and things that can be done in a group. Things that can be done alone include listening to the radio, watching television, reading, and doing skill games such as crossword puzzles, knitting, and painting. Things that can be done in a group include everything that can be done alone as well as playing cards, parties, and games.

The degree to which a patient can participate in recreation depends upon the nature of his illness, how quickly he tires, and his various abilities and interests. But no matter how limited or un-

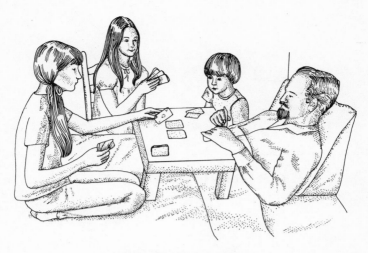

Family recreation with patient

limited his recreation time may be, at least part of it should be planned as social or group activity. For the very ill patient, this may mean something as simple as having a member of the family visit at mealtime and eat from a separate tray. For the more active patient it may mean a card game or a trip to the theater.

When caring for a patient at home, you should consider his particular interests. Perhaps he enjoys certain television programs, likes jigsaw puzzles, is a birdwatcher, and has for years played bridge every Tuesday night with a group of friends. To plan recreation for this patient you would arrange his treatments and routine so that he would be free to enjoy his favorite television programs. You would furnish interesting jigsaw puzzles and set aside a table for puzzle use only so he could work on a puzzle whenever he chose. You might have a bird-feeding station set up outside the window and arrange to take him, in a wheelchair if necessary, to areas where birds are commonly found. And by all means see that his bridge friends are invited to come on Tuesday evenings to play a few hands with him. If you don't play bridge, you might ask him to teach you the game.

Many kinds of recreational therapy are also useful as physical therapy. These include such activities as swimming, bird-watching or nature walks, and games such as shuffleboard.

5

Adaptive Equipment

Adaptive equipment is any article that allows a patient to regain use of a body part or to perform a body function.

Particularly as a patient ages and becomes less and less able to function, he becomes more and more dependent on adaptive equipment to keep him active and caring for himself. For mobility he may require special shoes as his first equipment; then a walking cane and an eating device; then a leg brace; next a walker; then a standard wheelchair, a different eating device, and an arm brace; and last, a special wheelchair. He nearly always needs glasses, and these are changed regularly to adapt to his failing vision. Often, he may require a hearing aid.

Two main kinds of adaptive equipment are used:

standard — manufactured alike but selected for size or adjusted to the size of the individual

custom — designed and made to suit the needs of the individual person

Certain general rules apply to the use of any adaptive equipment or devices.

Do not allow your patient to use a piece of equipment until he has been instructed in its safe and most effective use by a nurse or other professional instructor.

Know how to use a piece of equipment before helping your patient with its use.

Check every piece of equipment before and after use to determine its condition. If you cannot correct a defect report it to the mechanic who services the equipment, the visiting nurse, or the doctor. *Do not allow your patient to use a defective piece of equipment.*

Check any complementary equipment to determine its condition. EXAMPLE: Check the patient's shoes if he uses a walker, and report a defect that you cannot correct.

Keep the patient's personal equipment in his own room.

Place equipment so that the patient has easy access to it.

Take care of your patient's personal needs, such as toileting, before equipment is used.

See that the patient is dressed to allow the best use of the equipment.

Position the patient in the best manner to use the equipment.

See that the patient uses the equipment as instructed.

Allow him ample time to use the equipment by himself.

Observe his use of the equipment, and suggest changes for better use to the patient or visiting nurse.

During use of the equipment, check the patient's skin where it touches the equipment for indications of pulling or pinching from pressure.

Give special skin care before and after use of equipment to areas affected by use of equipment.

Report skin changes to the visiting nurse or doctor.

Do not allow a patient to exhaust himself through use of the equipment.

Clean the equipment after use.

Much adaptive equipment needs regular maintenance and repair. Specially trained mechanics are available through health services, medical supply houses, or some drugstores.

Arm Sling

An arm sling should not be used unless ordered by the doctor, except for temporary emergency treatment.

Equipment
    a triangle of heavy muslin
    two safety pins

Have the patient hold the affected arm in a natural and comfortable position, so that the upper arm rests against his side and the forearm crosses his waist.

Take the muslin triangle by one end of its longest side; hold the length straight up and down in front of the patient with the third corner directed toward the affected arm.

Slip the corner nearest the neck under the affected arm and to the back of the neck.

Bring the corner nearest the floor up over the affected arm and to the back of the neck.

Adjust these corners until the arm has snug, smooth support but is not lifted. The patient's hand should be slightly higher than his arm.

Tie the corners at the back of the neck but to one side of the spine. A knot on the bones of the spine causes pain and pressure.

Make a square knot to fasten.

Adjust the material under the length of the affected forearm so that the wrist and the hand are supported but the fingers are free and visible. Watch the fingers for signs of swelling or blue color. These signs indicate interference with the blood supply.

Adjust the material at the elbow to form a neat, snug corner and fasten with pins to the front of the sling.

Many commercial styles of arm slings are available and are often used. Read and follow the packaged instructions.

Artificial Replacements or Prostheses

A prosthesis is a device fitted to the body to replace a part that is missing. Artificial limbs, artificial eyes, and dentures are examples of external prostheses. Artificial femur heads, artificial blood vessels or heart valves, and cardiac pacemakers are examples of surgically implanted internal prostheses.

Cleanliness and daily care of an external prosthesis and the amputation or extraction site are of the utmost importance. The skin and membranes are easily irritated by contact with prostheses, and when an inflammation or rash occurs, use of a prosthesis may be suspended.

Helping the Patient with a Prosthesis

Report to the doctor if the patient complains of pain, pressure, or pinching from a prosthesis.

Check the prosthetic area before and after use for redness, rash, bruises, or swelling.

Check the prosthesis before and after use for loose, bent, broken, or stiff parts.

Report a defect of the prosthetic side of the patient or the prosthesis to the doctor at once.

IF THE PROSTHESIS IS A LEG OR AN ARM

Give special skin care before and after use of the prosthesis.

See that the patient has a supply of stump socks.

See that he wears a stump sock when using the prosthesis and afterward, except for airing periods. (Stump socks help to prevent swelling.)

Be sure that the stump sock is kept smooth and wrinkle-free to prevent creasing the skin.

See that the patient is dressed in clothes that allow easy use of the prosthesis. Trousers should be reinforced at the side where they contact a knee bolt and sleeves at the side where they rub against an elbow bolt. A cotton stocking should be worn under a nylon stocking to prevent runs due to the prosthesis.

Check stump socks for worn spots. Report such spots to the visiting nurse or doctor; worn spots indicate a need for correction of the prosthesis by a specialist.

Helping a Patient Put on a Leg Prosthesis

Equipment
   a stump sock
   the prosthesis
   a strong straight chair

Help the patient to a standing position, facing you.

Allow him to support himself by holding onto the back of a straight chair (the side of amputation should be closest to the chair).

See that the stump sock is clean, dry, and smooth. Draw it well up on the stump.

Place the prosthesis under the stump so that the toe is positioned outward.

Steady the prosthesis foot against the leg of the chair.

Push the stump into the socket.

Fasten the pelvic belt (this turns the toe of the prosthesis inward to a normal position).

Be sure the pelvic belt is horizontal and cannot ride up over the hip of the normal leg.

Smooth the sock at the top of the prosthesis.

Braces

A brace is an adaptive appliance used to support the body or a body part. A doctor always orders the use of a brace, and it is usually custom-made to fit a patient. A brace may be ordered to help a patient walk, to control involuntary body movements, and to correct and prevent deformity. Careful handling of a brace is essential to maintain correct brace alignment. You should also remember that such an appliance is expensive and that careful handling saves unnecessary expense.

The individual patient's use of a brace is affected by

his desire to walk;
his attitude toward the brace;
the comfort of the brace;
whether the brace is correctly applied.

A walking brace requires a special shoe to accommodate it, and both shoes and the brace should be inspected for signs of wear and need of repair before and after every wearing. It is best to leave the shoe attached to the brace.

The skin must be examined frequently for pressure areas caused by contact with a brace, and skin care should be given before and after each use of the brace. Signs of pressure should be reported to the visiting nurse or doctor immediately.

Clothing to be worn over a brace must be large and loose enough to accommodate the brace without strain. If the patient removes the brace during the day, it may be best for him to wear the brace outside of his clothing.

Encourage the patient to do as much as he can toward applying the brace by himself. Allow him ample time.

Applying a Short Leg Brace

Equipment
  lotion for skin care
  a sock or stocking

the brace
supportive shoes
a shoehorn

Position the patient lying or sitting in bed with legs extended.
Give skin care to areas that contact the brace. Check skin for signs of pressure.
Put on a sock or stocking that is free of holes or mends and that fits the foot without wrinkling.
Attach shoes to the brace, if necessary.
Tuck brace straps out of the way.
Slightly bend the patient's knee. Place the brace under the lower part of the leg, guiding the foot into the shoe and making sure that the patient's toes do not curl under.
Use a shoehorn, if necessary, to see that the heel is securely in the shoe.
Lace and tie the shoe securely.
Fasten the straps, allowing enough space to insert two fingers beneath the brace fastenings. If the brace has an ankle strap, fasten it around the outside of the opposite upright strip of metal.
Check the brace for signs of pressure on the leg.
Put the other shoe on the patient before helping him off the bed.

Canes

Good control of the body trunk and strength in the arm and hand are necessary for a patient to use a cane. A cane is ordered by the doctor to suit the need of the patient and is measured to suit that need. A patient needs a cane that serves one of two main purposes:

primarily to bear weight
primarily to maintain balance

If a cane is used primarily for weight bearing, it is carried on the same side as the weak leg. A cane for this purpose is measured so that the patient's arm is stiff when bearing down on the cane. When the patient walks, the cane is advanced, a step is made with the good leg, and weight is borne by the cane while the weak leg is brought forward.

If a cane is used primarily for balance, the cane is carried on the side opposite the weak leg. This cane is measured to allow for a

30-degree bend of the elbow. When the patient walks, the cane is moved forward before a step is made with the weak leg.

Two types of canes are common.

standard — a bent-handled cane available in several kinds of wood and aluminum

four-legged — an aluminum cane with a shovel type of hand-grip and four legs

Helping a Patient with a Cane

BEFORE USE

Check the patient's shoes for signs of wear or need of repair. Be sure the shoes fit well and are tied securely.

Check the cane tips and replace worn rubber suction tips. Clean tips if necessary.

Check the cane for loose screws, cracks, or splinters.

DURING USE

See that the patient stands as straight as possible and looks straight ahead, not at his feet.

See that he carries the cane on the side for which it is ordered.

A Loftstrand or Canadian crutch is often used as a substitute for a cane.

Corsets

A corset may be ordered for a patient if he needs support for his back or trunk or to help with a problem of balance.

Helping a Patient with a Corset

Give special skin care before and after use.

Inspect corset for broken, bent, or worn spots.

See that the corset is clean and dry.

See that a patient's bony areas are padded to prevent irritation from corset stays.

See that undergarments are worn over the corset to allow for easier use of the toilet.

Helping a Patient Put on a Corset

Equipment
  the corset
  padding material, if necessary (self-adhering foam is good)

Help the patient to lie on his side.

Roll under the far side of the corset halfway.

Place the roll against the patient's spine so that the middle two stays of the back of the corset support the spine. Position the corset low under the buttocks because it tends to ride up when the patient sits.

Tuck the rolled half of the corset under the patient's body.

Hold the corset in place while turning the patient onto his back.

Bring the ends of the corset together in front.

See that the sides are even and that the lower edge of the corset is placed just over the pubic bone.

Smooth the lower edge under the buttocks.

Fasten the corset, working upward from the lower edge and smoothing wrinkles from under the flaps.

Check the corset for correct space by inserting two fingers in the top of it when the patient is in a sitting position.

Crutches

A crutch or crutches may be ordered by the doctor for a patient after an amputation, fracture, operation, or an injury to a leg. Three types are common:

Loftstrand or Canadian. Usually custom-made, it fits the forearm by means of a metal cuff and is made of aluminum.

A patient is measured for a Loftstrand crutch by adjusting the cuff and handgrip so that his elbow is bent at about a 30-degree angle and the crutch tip extends from 6 to 8 inches to the side of his foot.

Loftstrand crutches are preferred because they allow a patient to adjust his clothes or to take hold of another object without losing the use of the crutch. They also eliminate the pressure on the ribs and arms that is unavoidable with an axillary crutch. They are often used instead of canes.

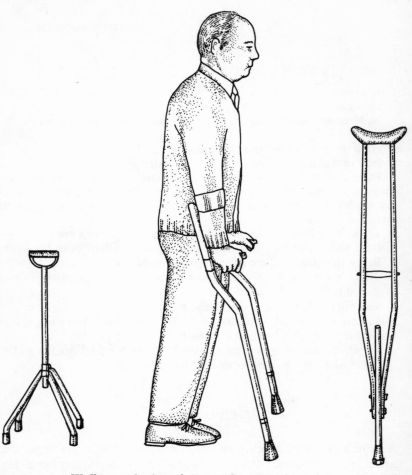

Walking aids: from left to right, a four-legged cane, a Lofstrand crutch, an adjustable crutch

Standard axillary. Nonadjustable, it fits into the patient's armpit and is usually made of wood.

Extension axillary. Adjustable, it fits into the patient's armpit and may be made of wood or aluminum.

A patient is fitted for axillary crutches by measuring the length from his armpit to a point 6 inches out from the side of the sole of his foot, or by measuring the length from his armpit to the side of the sole of his foot and adding 2 inches. The handgrips are adjusted so that the patient's elbows are bent at about 30-degree angles.

The axillary bar of a crutch is always padded to prevent undue pressure on ribs and arms.

Crutch Gaits

Four point. Move right crutch, left foot; left crutch, right foot. It is a simple, slow, but safe method; there are always three points of support on the floor.

Two point. Move right crutch and left foot simultaneously, then left crutch and right foot simultaneously. This requires more balance than the four-point method because only two points are supporting the body at any one time.

Three point. Move both crutches and the weaker lower extremity forward simultaneously and then move the stronger lower extremity forward. It is used when one lower leg cannot take full or any weight and the other leg can support the whole body weight.

Tripod alternate. Move right crutch, left crutch; drag feet forward. This method is used by those unable to lift either leg.

Tripod simultaneous (rockinghorse gait). Move both crutches forward simultaneously; drag feet forward. This method is also used by those unable to lift either leg.

Swinging to. Move both crutches forward; then lift and swing body forward just short of the crutches.

Swinging through. Move both crutches forward; then lift and swing body beyond crutches. Skill, strength, and proper timing are required. Use a swinging gait to lift the body off the floor when there is a severe disability of the lower extremities.

Sideward four point. Move right crutch to right; right foot to right; left foot to right; left crutch to right.

Backward four point. Move left foot back; right crutch back; right foot back; left crutch back.

Turning on crutches. Place one crutch in front of body, the other slightly to the side and rear; pivot feet or lift body in the direction crutches were moved. Repeat as often as necessary to make turn.

Helping the Patient with Crutches

BEFORE USE

Check patient's shoes for signs of wear or need of repair.

Be sure shoes fit well and are tied securely.

Check crutch tips and replace worn rubber suction tips. Clean tips if necessary.

Check crutch for axillary padding, loose screws, cracks, or splinters.

DURING USE

See that the patient stands straight and looks ahead, not at his feet.

See that he uses the crutch as taught.

AFTER USE

Check the body areas that contact the crutch for signs of pressure. Give special skin care to these areas.

Feeding Equipment or Devices

A feeding device is an appliance that is fitted to a hand or arm that has lost some function; it allows the patient to feed himself with little or no assistance. A patient with limited range of motion or muscle weakness might require such a device.

Patience is of the utmost importance when helping a patient with special feeding equipment. It may take him a long time to complete a meal, especially when he is just learning to use the device. Encourage him and allow him plenty of time to use the equipment, but do not let him become exhausted by his attempts or go hungry. Feed him if necessary.

Helping with Feeding Equipment

Equipment
   the patient's feeding device
   special silverware
   a plate guard to prevent spilling
   suction under the mat for holding the plate
   a rocker arm, overhead sling, or balancer
   special straws
   a bib or napkin

See that the patient is in a comfortable sitting position.

Place his arm in the rocker, overhead sling, or balancer if needed.

Put his bib or napkin around his neck.

Attach the feeding device and allow the patient a few practice swings with it to be sure he can reach both the plate and his mouth.

Position the food tray so that the patient has best access to it.

Prepare food, such as cutting meat or buttering bread, as necessary.

Put the food guard on the plate.

Be sure liquids are within the patient's reach.

Put straws in liquids.

Let the patient eat as independently as possible.

Give the patient sufficient time to eat, helping him if necessary.

Walkers

A walker offers a secure cage within which a patient can move without fear of falling. No patient should be allowed to use a walker unless a doctor has ordered its use. The walker is adjusted

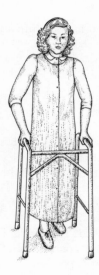

Using a walker

to the size and needs of the patient and he is instructed in its safe use. Elbows should be bent at 30-degree angles when the patient uses the walker. Three types of walkers are common:

Standard. A rigid four-legged frame used as an aid for balance and weight bearing when walking. It requires the use of safety suction tips. The patient's weight is thrown alternately to the front and back of the walker as he steps.

Gliding. A standard frame, adapted by putting button casters on the walker's metal tips. The patient is able to push the walker and still maintain good control. (Wheels on walkers have proved to be unsafe.)

Reciprocal. A hinged frame that allows the patient to move it forward one side at a time. It requires safety suction tips.

Helping the Patient Who Uses a Walker

BEFORE USE

Check the patient's shoes for signs of wear or need of repair.

Be sure the shoes are on correctly and are tied securely.

Check the walker tips and replace worn ones if needed. Clean the tips if necessary.

Check the walker for loose screws or defective parts.

DURING USE

See that the patient stands as straight as possible and looks ahead, not at his feet.

See that he uses the walker as taught.

Wheelchairs

Wheelchairs are ordered by the doctor for patients with a variety of handicaps, and many factors are considered in selecting the proper chair and accessories for the individual. The techniques of using a wheelchair also vary according to the individual patient's needs. The patient should not be allowed to use his wheelchair until he has been instructed in its use.

Universal. This chair has larger wheels in the back. It can be used indoors and outdoors; it ensures better posture, allows easier transfer activities, and can be tilted to go up curbs and stairs.

Traveler. This chair has larger wheels in front. It is only used indoors and on level surfaces; it allows poorer posture, is more difficult for transferring activities, and cannot be used for curbs or stairs.

Amputee. This chair has the rear wheels set back. It maintains safe balance by compensating for loss of the patient's weight in front due to amputation. Footrests and legrests are available for a one-sided amputee or a patient wearing a prosthesis.

One-arm drive. This chair has both handrims on one side. It may be prescribed for those who have only one good arm, such as the hemiplegic or the amputee. This chair is too wide for most doors, and it is difficult to learn to use.

Power-driven. This chair is propelled by a motor. It should be used only by patients with no other possible means of propelling themselves.

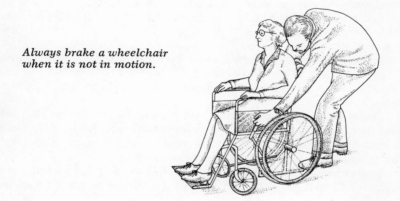

Always brake a wheelchair when it is not in motion.

Custom. This chair is designed for a specific patient.

Patients sometimes use two other kinds of wheelchairs. One is a small, strong, straight chair with caster wheels on the leg tips. It can be ordered in metal or adapted from a wooden kitchen chair. The other type is a commode wheelchair with an open seat and a removable waste pan for use by incontinent patients.

Wheelchairs are made in four sizes: adult; adult, extra wide; junior; child.

Wheelchair Accessories

A patient's disabilities and potential abilities determine which accessories are ordered for his wheelchair.

Brakes. Every wheelchair should be equipped with brakes for the patient's safety.

Wheels. Front casters that are 5 inches in diameter are standard equipment on wheelchairs; however, the 8-inch caster allows for better patient control. Handrims with multiple-grasp projections may be used by a patient who is unable to hold a regular handrim.

Armrests. Upholstered armrests allow greater comfort. Removable arms may be needed so that the patient can transfer in and out of the chair. Armrests may be equipped with button brake locks. Desk arms may be ordered if accessibility to a desk or table is necessary.

Backrests. Adjustable backrests may be ordered for the patient who is unable to sit in an upright position all the time. Zippered backrests may be ordered for a patient who must be transferred to and from the chair by being slid in and out of the back. Removable headrests may be ordered for additional back and head support.

Legrests. Adjustable legrests may be ordered for the patient who must have one or both legs elevated. Swinging detachable legrests may be ordered to allow the patient a closer approach in transferring.

Footrests. Heel loops, which prevent the feet from slipping off the footrest, may be ordered for one or both feet. A two-heel strap may be used if both feet must be held on the footrest. Toe loops for maintaining foot position may be ordered.

Seat cushions. Foam rubber seat cushions 2 to 4 inches thick are used for the patient's comfort and for prevention of pressure sores.

Care of Wheelchairs

Proper care of a wheelchair is important. Regular attention keeps a wheelchair in good condition and prolongs its usefulness.

Cleaning. Wipe all metal parts of the wheelchair once a week with a light coating of general-purpose household oil applied with a soft cloth. Wipe leather or plastic upholstery with a damp cloth and clean with saddle soap. Be sure to dry both chrome and leather whenever they are wet.

Lubrication. Oil the center bolt of the crossbars and the point of attachment of the brakes to the lower side bars. Grease both the front and rear wheel axles with petroleum jelly or any grease lubricant. (This is generally necessary only once a year.) Apply paraffin wax when needed to any telescoping parts, such as adjustable backs, removable arms, footrests, and extensions. *Do not oil or grease these parts.*

Miscellaneous. Be sure to keep nuts, bolts, screws, and other fastening devices tight; if any part breaks, have it repaired by an authorized wheelchair repairman. Be sure to use a wheelchair wrench for adjusting footrests.

Using a Wheelchair

A patient can manipulate a standard wheelchair by using both arms or by using one arm and one leg.

USING BOTH ARMS

Moving forward. Grasp the handrims as far toward the back of the wheels as possible and push both wheels forward at the same time. Long, even pushes are less tiring than short, erratic ones.

Turning. To turn a corner, push the wheel on the opposite side from the direction you want to turn and hold the other wheel still. To turn around in a small space, place one hand forward on one handrim and the other hand back on the opposite handrim; pull with the forward hand and at the same time push with the back hand.

USING ONE ARM AND ONE LEG

Moving forward. Pushing only one wheel turns the chair in a circle; therefore, push the wheel with the good hand and at the same time use the good foot to oppose and counter the turn and allow the chair to go forward.

Turning. To turn toward the affected side, use only the opposite hand to turn the wheelchair. To turn toward the unaffected side, reach across to the opposite wheel with the good hand and use the good foot in the same way as in the forward movement.

Helping the Patient with a Wheelchair

Keep the chair and pillow supports clean.

Inspect the chair before and after use for loose or improperly working parts.

Help the patient in transferring to and from the wheelchair.

See that the patient is positioned correctly in the chair and maintains good sitting alignment.

6

Feeding

Nutrition

Good nutrition means fulfilling the body's needs for certain elements. A proper diet prevents disease, gives energy, aids growth and repair of tissues, regulates the body's elimination, and stimulates appetite. Scientists have determined that the human body needs different amounts of the following:

proteins
carbohydrates
fats
vitamins and minerals
water

Protein foods are meat, fish, poultry, milk, cheese, and eggs. Protein builds, repairs, and maintains tissues. It is necessary for healthy hormone, enzyme, and blood function.

Carbohydrate foods are all starches (such as breads, flours, cereals, potatoes, rice), all sugars (such as table sugar, syrup, desserts, jellies, candies), and all fruits and vegetables (even though no sugar is added in their preparation). Carbohydrates give heat and energy, they help the growth of necessary intestinal bacteria, and give a sense of food satisfaction.

Fat foods are those that come from animals (such as meat trimmings, lard, butter, cream, egg yolk, and yellow cheeses) and those that are made from vegetable oils (such as corn, peanut, soya, cot-

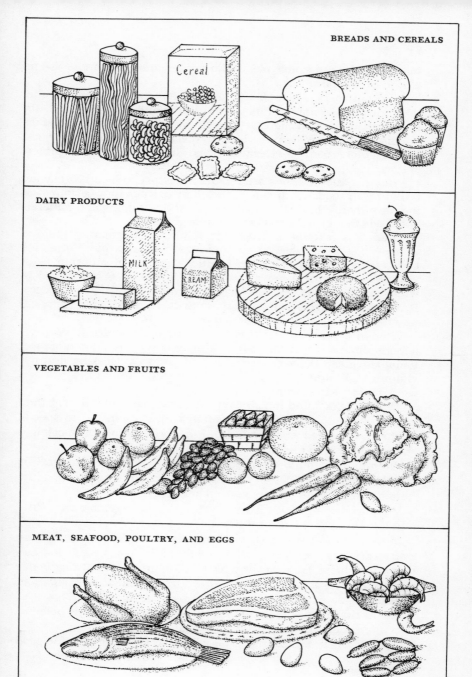

Food groups for good nutrition

tonseed, palm, and olive oils). Margarines and nut butters are included as vegetable fats.

In recent years, research studies have led doctors to believe that large amounts of animal fats are unhealthy and a general tendency has resulted to substitute vegetable oil for animal fat when possible.

Fats give energy, help the body to digest and utilize other foods, help regulate body temperature, and help support and protect organs.

Vitamins and *minerals* are factors necessary to health. They are found in all foods, with some foods being richer in a certain vitamin or mineral than others. Here is a list of vitamins and minerals and foods that give the richest amounts of them.

Vitamin A is found in liver, egg yolk, butter, cream, green and yellow vegetables, fish liver oil, and fortified margarine. Vitamin A is necessary for good vision and healthy bones, teeth, and skin.

Vitamin Bs (there are a number of B vitamins) are found in whole grains, meats, yeast, wheat germ, milk, liver, nuts, and eggs. B vitamins are needed for proper growth, healthy nerve function, and healthy digestion and elimination.

Vitamin C is found in citrus fruits (such as grapefruit, oranges, lemons, limes, tangerines). It is also in strawberries, cantaloupe, tomatoes, green peppers, cabbage, and potatoes. Cooking destroys vitamin C. Vitamin C helps fight disease, builds strong bones and teeth, and aids in enzyme function.

Vitamin D is found in fish liver oil, butter, egg yolk, liver, irradiated milk, and other foods. (*Irradiated* means exposed to special light rays that produce vitamin D). It helps the body utilize calcium and phosphorus in the formation of bones and teeth.

Vitamin E is found in wheat germ, leafy vegetables, vegetable oils, egg yolk, nuts, peas, and beans. Vitamin E helps in the healthy function of reproductive organs and hormones.

Vitamin K is found in leafy vegetables and vegetable oils. Vitamin K helps in the clotting of blood.

Minerals that are known to be necessary for body function are iron, iodine, copper, manganese, magnesium, potassium, and calcium. Iron helps build healthy blood. Calcium makes strong bones and teeth. Phosphorous helps growth and acid-alkaline regulation. Sodium regulates body fluids and acid-alkaline balance.

A diet that furnishes enough of the other necessities is believed to contain enough materials for a normal person.

In addition to a diet that gives all those foods needed for good nutrition, doctors often order additional vitamins and minerals to be taken in a pill or capsule. The pill or capsule may contain a mixture of many vitamins and minerals or a single vitamin or a combination of a few vitamins. The doctor's order depends on his evaluation of the needs of the individual patient.

Necessary foods are divided into four groups; for good nutrition a person should have the following amounts of foods from these groups every day:

DAIRY FOODS
    children — 3 to 4 glasses of milk
    teenagers — 4 or more glasses of milk
    adults — 2 or more glasses of milk

Cheese, ice cream, and other milk products can supply part of the milk.

MEAT
    two or more servings of meat, fish, poultry, eggs, or cheese.

VEGETABLES AND FRUITS
    four or more servings that should include dark green and yellow vegetables and citrus fruit or tomato.

BREADS AND CEREALS
    four or more servings.

Water, in addition to other fluids such as juice, is very necessary. Six to eight glasses daily are needed for a normal adult. Water helps maintain healthy fluid balance and helps rid the body of wastes.

Selecting and Preparing Foods

Talk to the patient about his food preferences and plan meals with these in mind or follow the specific diet ordered by the doctor.

Appeal to his senses. Select foods that look appetizing, smell good, and have different textures.

Select foods that furnish the patient's daily nutritional needs.

Cook foods in the simplest way. Bake, broil, boil, or steam them.

Cook vegetables quickly in a small amount of water. Save any liquid left in the pot after cooking, for it is rich in vitamins and minerals. Use this liquid in soups, vegetable drinks, or to cook other foods.

Avoid most fried foods, rich sauces, and heavy desserts. These foods tax digestion, decrease appetite, and do not give the best nourishment.

Remember that eating is a social occasion. Try to plan the family meal with the same foods as the patient requires and whenever possible have the family eat with the patient.

Many older people seem to lose their appetites and become disinterested in food. Many have small incomes. When they must shop for and prepare their own food, eating becomes a function that they are unable or unwilling to perform because of the effort and expense.

National and local governments and charitable organizations are taking an interest in the nutritional welfare of older citizens at home. Some organizations provide "meals on wheels." These are hot meals delivered once daily to older people. Other groups serve inexpensive hot meals to those over sixty-five in school, church, and social cafeterias. A few restaurants offer "senior citizen specials" or inexpensive daily nonchoice hot meals served during off-rush hours. You should learn what community services are available for older citizens and help your patient to benefit from them when possible.

Preparing a Tray for Service

Be sure the tray, dishes, silverware, and napkins are spotless.

Be sure sugar and salt containers are clean and filled.

Set the tray in careful order.

Serve small amounts of food unless you know the patient desires more.

Arrange the food in neat portions.

Serve hot foods hot and cold foods cold. Cover hot foods to keep them warm.

If possible serve one course at a time.

Preparing a Patient to Be Served

If the patient is restricted to bed care, offer a urinal or bedpan before mealtime.

Be sure the patient is in the most comfortable position for eating. If the patient feeds himself, be sure the tray is within easy reach.

Serving Food

Set the food before the patient so that he has the best access to it.
Encourage the patient to eat.
Observe how he uses adaptive equipment.
Help him to eat when necessary.

Feeding a Helpless Patient

Stand or sit beside the patient.
Take as much time as necessary and have a relaxed, pleasant attitude.

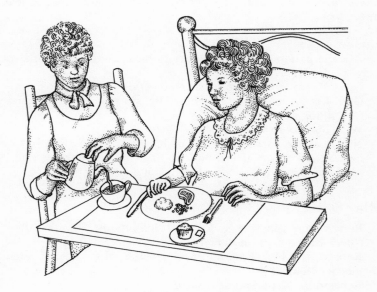

Sit and be comfortable when feeding a patient.

Encourage the patient to communicate his likes and dislikes.
Place a napkin or towel under the patient's chin.

GIVING LIQUIDS

Do not fill the glass or cup. Be sure the liquid is not too hot or too cold. Place one of your hands under the patient's pillow to raise his head. Hold the glass or cup in your other hand and let the patient control it.

If the patient cannot raise his head, turn his head toward you. Put a drinking straw into the liquid and insert the straw into the patient's mouth. Tell the patient to draw on the straw.

Always give liquids slowly.

If the patient is conscious but too weak to draw on the straw, handle the straw in the following manner. Hold the straw near the top between your thumb and third finger. Without bending the straw insert one end of it into the liquid. Place and hold your index finger over the top of the straw. This will hold the liquid in the straw. Insert the bottom of the straw into the lower corner of the patient's mouth. Remove your index finger from the top of the straw. Watch until the patient swallows and then repeat the procedure.

GIVING SOLIDS

Ask the patient if he would like to have the foods on his tray in any special order.

Use a fork or spoon to offer a small serving.

Give the patient time to chew. Be sure he swallows one bite before giving another.

Wipe his mouth when needed.

Notice and report how much of his meal the patient has eaten.

Notice and report if the patient has trouble chewing and swallowing any particular food or type of food.

After Eating

Remove any adaptive devices and clean them.

Check the devices for defects.

Remove the bib or napkin and see that the patient's face and hands are cleaned.

Reposition the patient as needed.

Diets

In caring for the sick, certain standard diets are used.

Clear Liquid Diet

Allows only clear broths, plain-flavored gelatins, clear tea, coffee, and carbonated drinks such as ginger ale.

Small amounts of fluids are offered about every two hours.

MEAL PLAN FOR A CLEAR LIQUID DIET
    8:00 A.M. coffee or tea
    10:00 A.M. ginger ale
    12:00 noon clear chicken broth, orange Jell-o
    2:00 P.M. tea
    4:00 P.M. mineral or carbonated water
    6:00 P.M. beef bouillon, raspberry Jell-o
    8:00 P.M. tea

A patient might receive a clear liquid diet after anesthesia, surgery, or a severe digestive upset.

Full Liquid Diet

Allows strained cream soups, thin cooked cereals, strained fruit juices, sherbets or vanilla ice cream, junket, custard, and milk added to the clear liquid diet. Small servings are offered every two hours.

MEAL PLAN FOR A FULL LIQUID DIET
    8:00 A.M. small glass strained orange juice, coffee, farina, milk
    10:00 A.M. beef broth
    12:00 noon strained cream of carrot soup, vanilla ice cream, tea with lemon
    2:00 P.M. apple juice
    4:00 P.M. chicken broth
    6:00 P.M. strained vegetable soup, custard, coffee with milk
    8:00 P.M. Jell-O, glass of milk

A patient might receive a full liquid diet as an in-between diet from clear liquid to soft diet, after dental surgery, or when a broken jaw has been wired for mending.

Soft Diet

Allows the following:

Breads: White, fine whole wheat, and seedless rye

Cereals: Dry; fine white, such as farina, Cream of Wheat, cornmeal, rice; strained coarse, such as oatmeal, Wheatena, grits

Crackers: White

Desserts: Custards; tapioca, rice, and bread pudding; sponge or angel cake, plain; frozen and gelatin desserts; cooked and canned soft fruit without seeds and skin, such as apricots, applesauce, peaches, pears, plums; ripe bananas, orange and grapefruit sections without membrane

Eggs: All ways except fried

Fluids: All liquids (except alcoholic) and strained soups

Meat: Tender meat (ground is best), poultry, fish

Milk and Cheese: Milk, soft cheese such as cream, cottage, and grated American in a sauce

Pasta: Plain noodles, spaghetti, and macaroni

Vegetables: Cooked asparagus, beets, carrots, peas, spinach, string beans, squash without seeds, mashed sweet potato, white potato without skin prepared any way except fried

AVOID: Coarse dark breads, whole-grain crackers, coarse dark cereals; rich pastries and any dessert with nuts, coconut, or fruits not on the allowed list; raw fruit except juice, ripe banana, orange and grapefruit sections; tough meat, gristle and meat fat, salted or smoked fish; spicy seasonings; raw, coarse, and strong-flavored vegetables.

MEAL PLAN FOR SOFT DIET

Breakfast
Soft fruit or fruit juice
Cereal with milk

Egg
Toast
Butter or fortified margarine
Coffee or tea

Luncheon or supper
Choice of soft cheese, tender meat, fish, poultry, or egg
Potato or substitute
Cooked vegetable
Bread
Butter or margarine
Fruit
Milk

Dinner
Tomato, orange, or grapefruit juice
Tender meat, fish, or fowl
Potato
Cooked vegetable
Bread
Butter or margarine
Dessert
Milk

Between-meal nourishment
Milk
Cocoa
Fruit juice

A patient might receive a soft diet if he were unable to chew, swallow, or digest a regular diet.

Bland Diet

This is the same as a soft diet but without seasonings, stimulants, or roughage. It is often given in frequent small feedings rather than meals.

MEAL PLAN FOR A BLAND DIET
Amounts should be about half average size.
8:00 A.M. strained orange juice or applasauce
Puffed Rice or farina with milk
decaffeinated coffee

10:00 A.M. beef bouillon
            white soda cracker
12:00 noon strained tomato or apricot juice
            poached egg or lean broiled ground meat
            mashed or baked potato without skin
3:00 P.M.   tea with lemon or milk
            ladyfinger
6:00 P.M.   broiled fish or breast of chicken
            creamed spinach or carrot puree
            gelatin salad with peeled canned fruit and cottage
                cheese
            decaffeinated coffee
8:00 P.M.   baked custard or rice pudding

A patient might receive a bland diet for certain disorders of the stomach and intestines.

Regular Diet

MEAL PLAN FOR A FULL, REGULAR, OR NORMAL DIET

Breakfast
Citrus fruit or juice
Whole-grain or enriched cereal with milk and sugar
Egg, cheese, or breakfast meat
Whole wheat toast
Butter or margarine
Coffee, tea, or cocoa with cream and sugar

Luncheon or supper
Cheese, meat, fish, or eggs
Potato or substitute
Vegetable
Salad with dressing
Whole wheat or enriched bread
Butter or margarine
Fruit (stewed or fresh)
Milk
Tea or coffee

Dinner
Soup or fruit or juice
Meat, fish, or fowl

Potato or substitute
Vegetable
Whole wheat or enriched bread
Butter or margarine
Dessert
Milk
Tea or coffee

Bedtime feeding
Milk, cocoa, or fruit juice may be given if the patient is hungry.

A patient would receive a regular diet if there were nothing in his condition to contraindicate it.

Between-Meal or Interval Nourishment

Avoid eating between meals unless snacks are a part of the diet plan. Nourishment in liquid form such as juice, milk, broth, tea, or coffee is preferred to solid foods for between-meal nourishment. Clear liquids do not interfere with the appetite and do help a patient maintain good fluid balance.

Special Diets

Doctors treat many diseases by exact regulation of the diet of an individual patient. Such a diet may deny the use of substances known to aggravate the illness or may increase the intake of foods which help improve the condition.

At home, a special diet is easily prepared from a diet sheet given by the patient's doctor. This sheet lists exactly what foods, and what amounts of each, the patient is allowed. It also tells what foods are forbidden. When your patient has a diet sheet, study it and follow it exactly.

Low-Salt or Low-Sodium Diet

Use no salt in cooking or preparing foods.
Use fresh vegetables and fruits.
Do not use any canned or frozen foods unless they are labeled *unsalted* or *salt-free*.

Do not use any packaged mix such as pancake, muffin, or cake mix.

Remove the salt shaker from the tray or table.

Use salt-free butter or margarine.

Do not use corned products such as beef or tongue.

Do not use frankfurters or luncheon meats or salted fish.

Do not use ready-to-eat cereals except Puffed Rice or Puffed Wheat.

Read food labels. The patient cannot have any sugar substitute that contains sodium. He can have saccharine if the doctor permits.

Be careful to check any diet drinks sweetened with sugar substitutes.

Use no pickles, relishes, jellies, or packaged gelatins and puddings.

Use unsalted bread and crackers.

Use no cheese except unsalted cottage cheese.

If eating in restaurants, the person on a low-sodium diet should limit himself to those foods to which no salt or monosodium glutamate (a seasoning) are added. These would include: milk, fresh fruit served whole (but not fruit cocktail or fruit salad, as monosodium glutamate is often added to these), boiled eggs, baked potatoes, broiled meats, fish, and chicken (if a special request is made for them to be prepared without salt).

SAMPLE LOW-SALT DIET

Breakfast

Fresh orange juice

Hot cereal cooked without salt

Boiled egg or unsalted cottage cheese

Toasted unsalted bread

Unsalted margarine

Honey

Tea or coffee with sugar or saccharine and milk or cream

Lunch

Chicken breast (boiled or broiled without added salt)

Fresh squash (cooked without salt)

Tossed fresh green salad with oil and fresh lemon juice dressing

Unsalted melba toast or matzos crackers

Unsalted margarine

Tea or coffee with sugar or saccharine and milk or cream

Dinner

Broiled or baked meat or fish (prepared without added salt)

Fresh spinach (cooked without salt)

Baked potato or boiled rice (cooked without salt)

Salad of lettuce and sliced fresh tomato with oil and vinegar dressing (no added salt)

Unsalted bread and unsalted margarine

Fresh sugared strawberries

Sponge cake (made without salt)

Whipped cream

Coffee or tea with sugar or saccharine and milk or cream

Certain vegetables and fruits have a high natural salt content. Sometimes the doctor will order these vegetables and fruits restricted.

One of the most common complaints about a low-salt diet is that the food is tasteless. This can be overcome to a certain extent by preparing foods, such as vegetables, by quick-cooking methods, using lemon juice at the table instead of a salt shaker, and by preparing foods with a variety of textures. EXAMPLE: Boiled potato, boiled carrots, and a slice of fresh bread have very similar textures. Baked potato, raw carrot strips, and toast have different textures.

Sodium-free salt substitutes are available at health food stores but should be used only with the doctor's permission.

Low-Cholesterol (Animal Fat) Diet

Use only vegetable oils or margarine in food preparation and at the table. Do not use butter.

Limit egg yolk intake. The doctor will indicate how many eggs a week the patient may have. Notice must be taken of eggs used in cooking; these yolks count too. Such foods as sponge cake and mayonnaise prepared with egg yolks should not be served.

Trim all fat from meat and poultry and use cuts of meat that have less fat. EXAMPLE: Round steak has much less fat marbling than sirloin.

Do not use ready-ground hamburger. Ask the butcher to grind a piece of completely fat-trimmed round steak instead.

Do not use any cheeses except cottage cheese made from skim milk.

Do not use whole milk, cream, or desserts that use whipped cream.

Skim or fat-free milk may be used.

Do not use meat gravies.

Do not use luncheon meats or canned meat spreads.

Do not use bread, cakes, or pies that use whole milk or butter or lard in their preparation. (Read the label.)

Do not use canned or frozen soups or other foods that contain meat, milk, or chicken fats.

SAMPLE LOW-CHOLESTEROL DIET

Breakfast

Fresh fruit or juice

Hot cereal with skim milk and sugar or saccharine

Toast with margarine and jelly

Coffee or tea with skim milk or nondairy lightener

Lunch

Broiled fish filet seasoned with margarine

Spinach (cooked in a plain manner and without cream sauce)

Mashed potatoes (use skim milk and margarine to prepare)

Green salad with oil and vinegar dressing

Water roll and margarine

Fruit gelatin with nondairy topping (read the label)

Coffee or tea with nondairy lightener

Dinner

Baked chicken (remove all skin and fat from chicken before cooking)

Curried rice (a packaged mix can be used)

French string beans

Angel food cake

Canned peaches

Coffee or tea with nondairy lightener

Between-meal nourishments of fruit juice, fresh fruit, or skim milk can be used.

Low-Calorie Diet

Prepare all vegetables by quick-cooking methods.

Do not season with butter, salt, oil, cream sauces, or gravies.

Roast, broil, or boil all meat, fish, or poultry.

Remove all fat and skin from meat or poultry before preparing.

Restrict use of bread, cereals, and sugar. Use saccharine if the doctor permits.

Do not use pies, cakes, ice cream, sour cream, whipped cream, cream, whole milk, cheeses (except for skim-milk cottage cheese), fruits canned in heavy syrup, candy, etc.

Do not use beans, corn, spaghetti, or other pastas.

SAMPLE LOW-CALORIE AND LOW-FAT DIET

Breakfast
Half a grapefruit without sugar
Boiled egg
One slice protein bread without butter or margarine
Coffee or tea with skim milk or lemon and saccharine

Midmorning
Cup of low-calorie broth

Lunch
Large tossed salad of greens, tomatoes, cucumbers, green pep-per, etc. Use low-calorie commercial dressing or, if re-stricted in use of salt, one tablespoon of vegetable salad oil, herbs, and lemon juice
Two pieces of melba toast
A glass of skim milk

Midafternoon
A small apple

Dinner
Small serving of broiled lean fish, meat, or poultry
Two large helpings of cooked vegetables such as green beans, squash, celery, tomatoes, cabbage, Brussels sprouts, broc-coli, spinach, collards, mustard greens, turnip greens, wax beans, asparagus
One small baked potato without margarine or sour cream
Cole slaw (made without mayonnaise, oil, or cream)
Slice of melon
Tea or coffee with saccharine and skim milk

Bedtime
A glass of skim milk or a small piece of fruit

Fluid Balance

Fluid balance means that the amount of liquid put out by the body balances the amount taken in. Many conditions can upset this balance.

Measuring Fluid Intake

Restoring or maintaining the balance can be difficult. Then the doctor wants to know exactly how much fluid is taken in and put out by the patient each day.

The average daily fluid intake for the normal adult of medium size is three quarts, or 3,000 cc.

A normal output would be about 250 cc. (or half a pint) less. That would be 2,750 cc.

Fluid, or liquid, is usually taken in orally. Fluid intake includes anything that the patient drinks or that dissolves to liquid if taken in his mouth. Water, milk, eggnog, milk shake, malted milk, juice, soup, broth, tea, coffee, soda, beer, ice cream, ice sherbet, junket, and gelatin are all counted.

Sometimes fluid is taken in through a vein. Intravenous, or IV, fluids include blood, plasma, normal saline solution, and dextrose water.

On occasion, fluid intake may result from a retention enema or from fluid injection under the skin.

Regardless of the way it is taken in, a record must be kept of the time, amount, and method of entry of any fluids taken. All IV fluid intake is totaled at the end of each twenty-four hours. All oral fluid intake is totaled at the end of each twenty-four hours. All retained rectal fluid intake is totaled at the end of each twenty-four hours. All skin injection fluid of more than 5 cc. is totaled at the end of each twenty-four-hour period. Then these totals are added to get the patient's fluid intake for that day.

When a patient is on measured intake, an intake sheet and pencil may be taped to the patient's bedside table.

Mark down on this sheet the fluid and amount taken whenever you remove any glass, pitcher, cup, dish, container, or tray from the bedside of the patient on measured intake.

7

Handling

It is easier for you and more comfortable for the patient if you follow these general rules for handling.

Tell the patient what you intend to do.

Don't place your hands on a pressure area or incision.

If the patient has painful joints, do not take hold of a joint, but grasp the arm or leg above or below the joint.

If the patient has painful muscles, do not take hold of the muscles, but grasp the joint.

Whenever possible, get the patient to help you.

Positioning

Illness affects the balance and strength of a patient. He may be dependent on your help to position himself in bed or a chair, to lift himself from a lying to a sitting position, and to transfer himself from bed to a chair or wheelchair.

For bedridden patients who have problems with moving about in bed, a routine of regular turning should be carried out. Such a routine is usually scheduled every two hours during an entire twenty-four-hour day. When possible, a patient is turned from one side to back to the other side and then onto his stomach.

Support can be given to hips, knees, shoulder, and other body parts by using pads, pillows, rolled towels, or rolled cotton blankets.

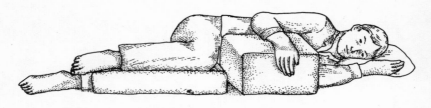

Side bed positioning, using pillows to align body parts.

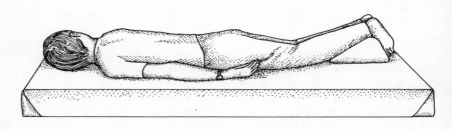

Stomach bed positioning, using pillow to maintain feet in neutral position.

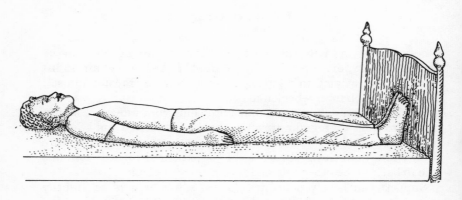

Correct backlying position.

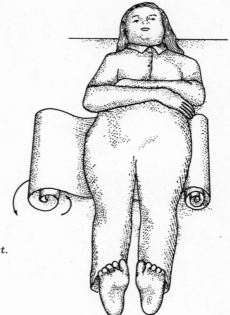

*Supporting legs
with a rolled cotton blanket.*

Preventing Legs from Rotating

With sandbags: Sandbags can be placed along the sides of the leg (from hip to knee) to keep the leg from rotating.

With a cotton blanket roll: A blanket roll may be used to prevent legs from rotating outward.

Positioning the Patient in a Chair

The way you position and support a patient to sit in a chair is very important. It can make the difference between his comfort and desire to sit and his fatigue, pain, and unwillingness to sit.

Keep the patient's spine straight and his body in line.

Place the lower part of his back against the back of the chair so that the body weight is equally distributed between thighs and buttocks.

See that his lower legs are at right angles to thighs.

Place his feet flat.

Correct body sitting position.

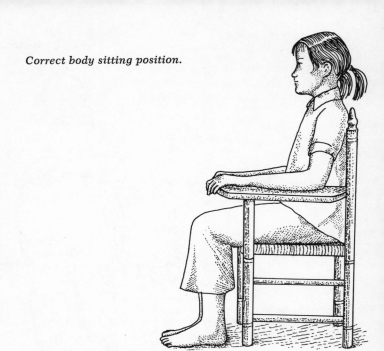

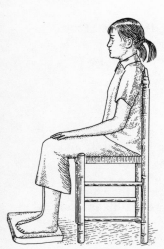

When seat is too high correct with a pillow under feet.

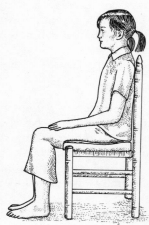

When seat is too short correct with a pillow on seat.

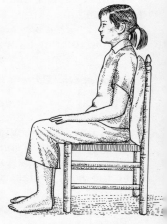

When seat is too long correct with a pillow at back.

Place his arms on armrests so that they are supported and help maintain body balance.

Use pillows and footstools to correct sitting alignment.

USING SAFETY EQUIPMENT

Sometimes, for the safety of the patient, it is necessary to use a belt or chest restraint that will hold him in the chair. These should be put on so that they maintain body alignment and do not interfere with a patient's blood circulation or comfort.

Lifting and Moving

Whenever you have a choice, always move your patient from side to side by sliding or rolling instead of lifting.

Always position your patient so as to get the best possible help from him.

Even the most helpless patient can help some if you do the following:

Put the mattress flat.

Remove any pillows.

Position the patient on his back and as close to you as possible.

Raise his knees so that the bottom of his feet are slightly apart and rest flat on the bed.

Bend your knees and hips and use your thigh and arm muscles rather than your back.

Always get help if the patient is very heavy.

How to Stand When Lifting and Moving a Patient

Stand erect. There is an easy trick to this. Keep your knees bent very slightly. This forces your shoulders back, tightens your stomach muscles, tucks in your hips, and cradles the weight of your body in the pelvis, or strong circle of bone above the hips.

Wear comfortable low-heeled shoes.

When lifting or moving a patient, stand as close to him as possible. Stand flat with feet apart. Point your toes in the direction of intended movement.

Lifting a Bed Patient to a Sitting Position

Follow the general rules for handling and for moving and lifting.

Have the patient lie with his legs extended.

Have the patient reach under your nearest arm and grasp your shoulder with his nearest hand.

Reach under the patient's nearest arm and grasp his shoulder.

Lock the arms together.

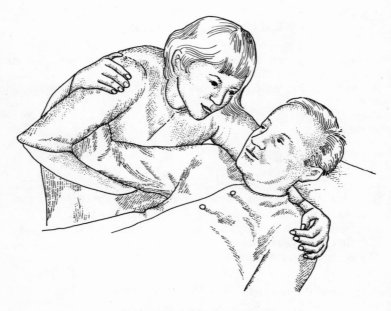

Helping patient sit up in bed

Bend and reach your upper arm under the patient's head and shoulders so that his head rests on your forearm and your hand grasps his far shoulder.

Avoid breathing in the patient's face.

Pull back to lift the patient.

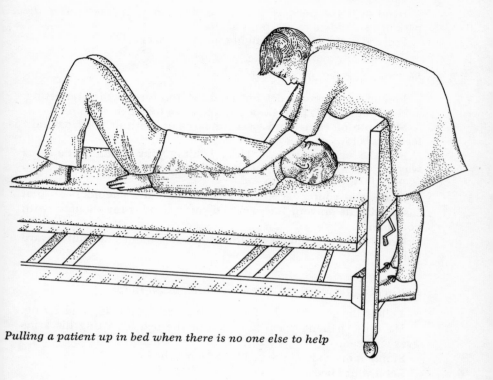

Pulling a patient up in bed when there is no one else to help

Pulling a Patient Up in Bed

Follow the general rules for handling and for moving and lifting.
Have the patient bend his knees and dig the soles of his feet against the mattress.
Place your upper arm to support his head and shoulders and your other hand to support his hips.
Pull the patient up to a count of three.

Pulling a Helpless Patient Up in Bed

Follow the general rules for handling and for moving and lifting.
Pull the bed away from the wall.
Lock the wheels of the bed.
Stand behind the head of the bed.
Climb onto the leg brace of the bed or onto a small stool.

Bend over the head of the bed and reach your hands over the patient's shoulders to grasp his armpits.

Pull the patient up by straightening your back.

Sliding a Bed Patient Nearer

Follow the general rules for handling and for moving and lifting.

Hold your hands palms upright and close together.

Slip both of your hands well underneath both of your patient's legs just below his knees.

Pull the legs toward you. Then, holding your hands in the same way, slip them well under the patient's hips.

Pull the hips toward you.

Then, slip your near arm under the patient's shoulders so that his head rests on your forearm and you grasp his far shoulder with your hand.

Grasp his near shoulder with your other hand and pull toward you.

Pulling Up the Mattress When the Patient Can Help

Follow the general rules for handling and for moving and lifting.

Have the patient grasp the head of the bed by lifting his arms over his head.

Stand at one side of the bed half-facing the head.

Bend your knees.

Take hold of the mattress loops.

On a count of three, you and the patient pull upward together.

Pulling Up the Mattress When the Patient Cannot Help

Follow the general rules for handling and for moving and lifting.

Two people stand one on either side of the bed.

Both take hold of mattress loops.

They pull upward together on a count of three.

Using a Drawsheet to Roll and Lift the Patient

Follow the general rules for handling and for lifting and moving.

Fold a drawsheet in quarters and lay it beneath the patient so that it is under his body from the shoulders to the thighs.

To turn the patient toward you, face the side of the bed and

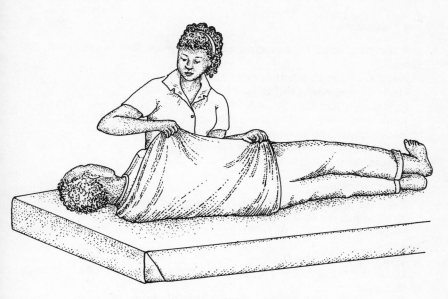

Using a drawsheet to roll a patient in bed

grasp the far edges of the drawsheet near the patient's shoulder and hip, then pull the sheet to you.

The quartered drawsheet may also be used by two people to pull a very heavy person up in the bed.

Follow the general rules for handling and for moving and lifting.

Lifters stand on both sides of the bed and face each other.

Each lifter grasps the quartered drawsheet at the patient's shoulder and hip.

On a count of three they pull the drawsheet upward.

Changing a Patient's Pajamas in Bed

BUTTON TOP (A slipover top is not recommended)

Roll the patient onto his far side.

Unbutton the top that the patient is wearing.

Remove his arm from the sleeve.

Undertuck the removed portion of the top between the patient's back and the mattress.

Reach inside from the cuff to the shoulders of the correct sleeve of the clean pajama top.

Take hold of the patient's hand and draw the sleeve over the arm.

Adjust the top in position on the shoulder and back.

Undertuck the remaining part of the top.

Roll the patient onto his near side.

Remove the soiled shirt from that arm.

Reach inside the sleeve and take the patient's hand.

Draw the sleeve onto the arm.

Adjust the top and button it.

PANTS

Keep the lower part of the body covered by a sheet.

Ask the patient to hold the top edge of the sheet.

Have the patient lie flat with knees bent and soles flat against the bed.

Working under the sheet:

Undo the waist of the pajamas and push the body of the pajamas to the hips.

Use one hand to help the patient to lift his hips for a minute.

At the same time, use the other hand to withdraw the pajamas from the buttocks.

Allow the patient to relax his buttocks.

Push the legs of the pajamas down to the ankles.

Lift one ankle at a time to remove the pants.

Reach inside from the foot to the top of the far leg of the clean pajamas and take hold of the patient's far foot.

Lift the foot and draw the pant leg onto the ankle.

Replace the foot on the bed.

Put on the other pant leg in the same way.

Draw both pant legs over the patient's legs to his buttocks.

Use one hand to help the patient lift his buttocks and use your other hand to draw the pants over the buttocks.

Allow the patient to relax his buttocks.

Straighten and adjust the pant leg and fasten the waist.

Teaching the Patient to Help Himself Turn and Sit Up

You can teach a patient how to turn himself by using a side rail. Have him lie on his back with knees flexed and grasp the rail with his far hand. Then he can pull himself over.

You can teach a patient how to raise himself to a sitting position by pulling on a length of rope tied securely to the center footstead of the bed.

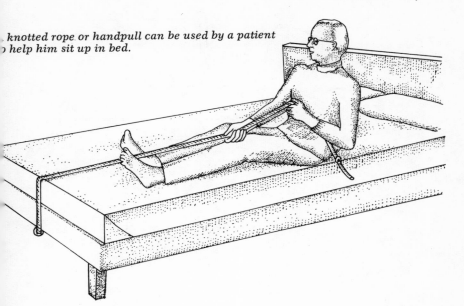

knotted rope or handpull can be used by a patient
to help him sit up in bed.

Using a Board to Transfer a Patient from Bed to Chair

Equipment
> a length of strong board, such as shelving, which has been
> sanded smooth and polished (can be acquired from a local
> carpenter)

Position the bed or chair seat to the same level.

Allow patient to sit up with legs over the bedside and feet touching floor.

Position chair or wheelchair at an angle facing the bed and patient.

Lay one edge of the board alongside the patient and the other edge on the chair to form a bridge. Be sure the bridge is secure.

Allow the patient to slide himself onto and along the board by using his arms and feet to steady and move his body.

Patient Transfer from Bed to Wheelchair

Have the patient sit on the side of bed with his legs dangling.

Place the wheelchair at an angle facing the bed and as close to it

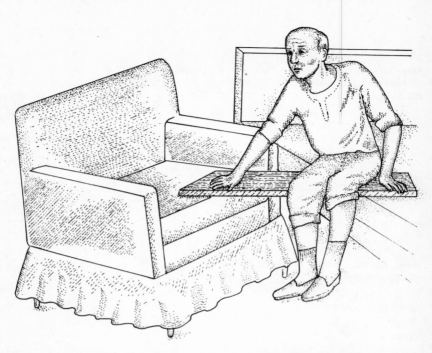

A patient using a board to transfer from bed to chair

as possible so that the patient's legs are between the bed and the chair.

Lock the wheelchair brakes.

Have the patient place the hand that is closest to the wheelchair on its far armrest and place his other hand on the bed and close to his buttocks.

Have him lift and pivot into the wheelchair, bearing most of his body weight on his hands and arms.

This method is used in reverse to transfer from the wheelchair to the bed.

Patient Transfer from Wheelchair to Straight Chair

Position the wheelchair so that the footrests straddle one front leg of the chair.

Lock the wheelchair brakes.

Have the patient slide forward to the edge of the wheelchair and place his nearest hand on the seat and his other hand on the arm-rest.

Have him lift and pivot himself, bearing most of his body weight on his arms.

This method is used in reverse to transfer from the straight chair to the wheelchair.

This method may also be used to transfer to a lower bench or toilet.

Transferring the Patient with a Mechanical Lifter

A mechanical lifter can move a helpless or a very fat patient with safety and ease. Lifters such as Hoyer or Porta-lift are designed to lift and hold much heavier weights than any patient. Some lifters have adjustable base widths to allow for passage through doorways. The base of a lifter should always be wide enough to prevent tipping during lifting. Lifters are operated by a hand pump. A lifter is used to transfer a patient from a bed to a chair or a commode and from a wheelchair into an automobile.

Since a patient may be fearful when using a lifter for the first time, its operation should be explained to him and every effort made to calm his fears. Two attendants helping at that time may ease his anxiety.

Slings and harnesses should be clean, comfortable, and in safe condition.

TRANSFERRING THE PATIENT FROM BED TO CHAIR
Equipment
    a lifting machine
    a canvas back and seat slings (Adjust slings to the individual
        and mark adjustment points for the patient. For example,
        mark the particular chain link with a string.)

Explain to the patient what you are going to do.
Place the patient on his back in a supine position.
Turn the patient as necessary to position the back and seat slings. Be sure that the seat sling is under the lower part of his buttocks and above the bend of his knees.
Bring the lifter close to the bedside.
Attach the S hooks (suspended by chains from the lifter) to the back and seat slings.
Shut the release knob.
Pump the handle to raise the patient above the mattress.

Check the patient and machine for good balance.

Swing the patient's feet off the bed.

Use the guide handles to move the patient away from the bed.

Suspend the patient directly over the chair, commode, or other object onto which he is to be placed.

Slowly open the release knob and lower the patient into the chair or other object.

When patient is seated, disconnect the S hooks.

Do not remove the sling supports. Leave them in place on the patient until he has been returned to bed.

SPECIAL SAFETY RULES

If the patient is very thin or has pressure sores, protect pressure points with extra padding.

Protect the patient against skin injury from the S hooks.

Always watch and protect the patient's legs and feet. Never allow them to bump against furniture or wheelchair rests.

Three-Person Carry

Rearrange furniture to allow sufficient space for turning and transferring.

Level the mattress.

Protect pressure areas with self-adhering foam.

Position the patient on his back with his arms either crossed over his chest or extended along each side.

Position the stretcher or table at a right angle to the foot of the bed on the side of the persons who will be lifters. The head of the stretcher should be near the bed.

Three people stand side by side and face the side of the bed from which the patient is to be lifted.

The second person counts and controls the motions.

FIRST PERSON

He supports the patient's head and shoulders with one arm and places his other hand and arm under the patient's body, just below the waist. (A small pillow under the patient's head can be included in this hold.)

SECOND PERSON

He places one arm under the patient's back, crossing it beneath the arm of the first person to support the patient's chest. He places his other hand and arm under the patient to support the thighs at the hip.

THIRD PERSON

He crosses one arm over the second person's arm to reach under and support the entire buttocks. He places his other arm under both calves.

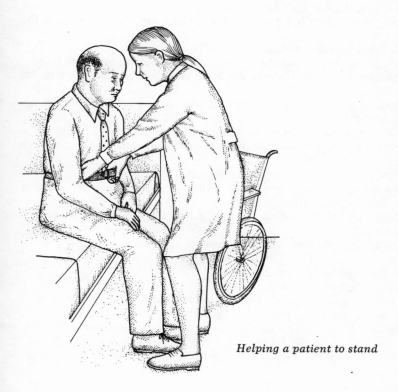

Helping a patient to stand

PROCEDURE

The second person counts to three.
On the count of one, the three people secure their holds.
On the count of two, the three people bend their knees.
On the count of three, the people lift together.
On the count of four, the people step back.

On the count of five, the people turn toward the stretcher at the foot of the bed and walk toward it.

On the count of six, they deposit the patient on the stretcher.

Transferring a Helpless Patient to a Wheelchair or Chair

Dress the patient.

See that he is wearing a belt or clothing with a strong waistband.

Position the wheelchair.

Help the patient to sit with his legs dangling over the side of the bed.

Position his body as close to the edge as possible.

Ask the patient to relax his body and not to try to help you.

Position his arms close to his body with his hands folded in his lap.

Position his feet together and aligned under his body. Point his toes forward.

Face the patient and straddle his legs.

Position your feet so that they brace the outsides of the patient's feet.

Squeeze your legs to brace the patient's legs.

On the side toward which you will be turning, place the palm of your near hand on the patient's hip.

Grasp the center of the patient's belt or waistband with your other hand.

Then make the following movements at the same time:

Pull on the belt or waistband.

Straighten your back.

Lock the patient's knee, on the side toward which you are turning, by pressing your knee against the patient's kneecap.

Swivel the patient's buttocks toward and into the chair.

8

Bed, Bed Equipment, and Bedmaking

Any patient spends more time in bed than a healthy person, so thought should be given to making the bed comfortable and convenient for the patient and for those who take care of him.

When a standard house bed is used for giving patient care, it can be adapted to suit patient needs in several ways.

Backrest

A backrest can elevate the patient's back to support a sitting position. Commercial backrests are available from medical or sleeping aids supply houses. A straightback, armless chair can be upturned and placed at the head of the bed between the bedboard and the mattress so that the patient's back rests against the chair back.

Bed Board

Placing a bed board between the springs and the mattress makes a firm surface for the patient to lie on that allows better body positioning, better blood circulation, and easier attendance by another to the patient. A bed board is a hinged (to fold double) lightweight board that is the size of a single mattress when unfolded. A bed board can be purchased from a medical or sleeping aids supply house or drugstore.

Bedtray

A bedtray for eating, writing, or a similar use can be obtained from a medical or sleeping aids supply house. One can also be made from a large, strong, rectangular cardboard grocery box. Use one with a firm bottom that has been opened only from its top.

Cut off the top flaps.

Strengthen the box by inserting another cut-to-size piece of cardboard in the bottom.

Cut out smaller identical-sized rectangles from the two long sides of the box.

Invert the box. It should fit over the patient's legs without restraining them. To make a smoother top surface, cover the top with Contak paper.

Bedcradle

A bedcradle, for holding covers off of an injured, burned, or infected part of the body, is available in different sizes and materials such as metal or plastic from medical supply houses. One can also be made from a strong cardboard grocery box of the correct size to fit over the specific body part (arm, thigh, foot). It is made in the same way as the bedtray (see above). When used as a cradle, rows of holes should be punched in the box to allow for better air circulation and for tying the box in position over the part.

Protective Drawsheets

A piece of plastic three feet wide and long enough to fit crosswise on the bed and tuck well under the mattress on both sides can be used as a mattress protector. On the bed, the plastic drawsheet is covered with a four-foot-wide and equally long piece of sheeting (two or more of these can be made from one old full-sized bedsheet). The cloth protective drawsheet can be changed as frequently as necessary or as desired without changing the entire bottom sheet. These sheets make it possible to keep a clean, dry, wrinkle-free surface under the patient without excessive discomfort, work, or laundry.

Protective Sides

Protective sides to prevent a patient from falling out of the bed can be made by moving the bed so that one side is against a wall. Then, place one or more chairs against the open side of the bed so that the chair backs rail the bed.

Bed Waste Bag

A waste disposal container for the bed can be made from a large brown paper grocery bag. Cut off the upper half of one side of a bag. Tuck the long upper side under the mattress. This leaves an exposed packet handy for used tissues, etc.

Bed Handy

A similar but larger container to hold useful items such as eyeglasses, pencil and pen, writing paper, tissues, a nail file, and the like, can be made from a strip of strong cloth. Sew a pocket on one end of the cloth. Leave a long free end to tuck under the mattress. If desired, the pocket can be sewn into dividers that fit the special items.

Hospital Beds

Hospital beds are available on a rental basis from medical supply houses.

Handcrank

This is a waist-high bed with two handcranks at the foot. The upper portion of the bed is raised or lowered by turning one crank; the knee area of the bed is raised or lowered by the other.

Electric

The electric bed is operated when buttons are pushed on a hand control box. The operation is so easy that the patient positions himself when that is desirable. This bed offers more positioning possibilities. As well as elevating the back and knees, the entire bed level can be raised or tilted headward or footward. Hospitals that use electric beds usually have a safety policy. A bed must be kept in low position at all times except when someone is with the patient. Slide rails are a part of the bed; these raise and lower by an easy-to-operate hand control.

Fracture

This is the usual hospital bed to which has been added some special equipment. For a person in a heavy body cast, a trapeze is attached to the bed in such a way that it hangs securely within the patient's upreached grasp. If the patient pulls on the trapeze, he can help move himself about the bed.

Traction

When a doctor wishes to stretch a certain part of a patient's body, he will order traction applied to that part. Then special frames are attached to a bed so that the affected part of the body is put in an outstretched position and pulled by heavy weights.

Footboard

A footboard is often used on the bed of a patient who suffers from arthritis, stroke, diabetes, heart disease, kidney disease, or any other condition that can cause foot trouble.

A footboard is a removable, smooth-surfaced board that can be placed between the bottom edge of the mattress and the footstead of the bed. It prevents top bed covers from pressing on the patient's feet. It also keeps the patient's feet in a neutral position because the soles rest flat against the surface of the board. This prevents foot deformity.

Footboards of various materials and several styles are available from medical supply houses. In a home situation, one can be improvised from a cardboard box, a dresser drawer, or a similar object. The best type, however, can be easily made by a local carpenter. It is made from two equal pieces of ½-inch plywood cut 10 inches shorter than the width of the mattress. The width of the boards is the sum of 2½ inches plus the length of the patient's feet, plus the thickness of the mattress. The boards are joined at right angles and the angles reinforced by two 3½-inch cubes of wood attached one to each side.

When put on the bed, this footboard holds very securely. One half fits the mattress so that the mattress edge rests against the cubes. The other half fits the footstead. A special advantage of this kind of footboard is that the patient can be placed on his abdomen with his feet extending beyond the edge of the mattress and the board will hold his feet in a neutral position.

Bedding

A mattress should be firm, not lumpy.

Old sheets that have softened from many washings are less irritating to the skin than new sheets. Lightweight blankets are more comfortable than heavier ones. Thermal blankets are particularly good for the sick bed since they are light, warm, and easily washed. Strong detergents or bleach should be avoided when washing bedding for a sick bed because they are irritating to the skin. A very light starching of bedsheets and ironing can make them smoother and more comfortable for a patient.

Pillows are largely a matter of individual choice. However, one firm and one soft head pillow allow for more head positioning possibilities. A number of other pillows of various sizes should be available for the positioning of bedridden patients.

A sheet can be used as a spread to cover the blanket of a bedridden patient.

Bedbugs

A flatish, oval, red-black insect that lives in neglected houses, furniture, and beds. It feeds on human blood and is active at night.

Signs of bedbugs are: night itching, skin rashes showing a typical pattern of three-in-a-row bites.

The best care is prevention through cleanliness of self, bed, and house. When infestation occurs, disinfect all infected areas. Professional extermination may be needed for house or furniture infestation. Careful washing and spraying of disjointed bed parts and the mattress will usually clear out a mild infestation. Various brands of specific insecticides are available from supermarkets and drugstores.

Bed Restraints (Wrist and Ankle)

Restraints are used only when a doctor orders them, except when the patient is in danger of harming himself or others. Then restraints may be put on until the doctor is notified of the patient's condition. REMEMBER:

If one wrist is restrained, the other must also be restrained.

If feet are restrained, wrists must also be restrained.

Before Applying Restraints

Be sure the patient is in a normal comfortable position.

Bathe the wrists and ankles with warm water.

Dry them well.

Rub them with skin lotion.

Pad them with cotton or foam rubber.

Never fasten restraints so tight that the patient cannot move his limbs.

After Applying Restraints

Watch for skin changes that indicate the blood supply is shut off. White, blue, gray, or cold skin is a sign of poor blood circulation. If such signs occur, remove the restraints.

Check the restraints at regular intervals.

Remove them every four to six hours and repeat skin care.

After removing, repeat skin care.

Using a Length of Material as a Restraint

Make a restraint knot in the center of the strip of material (see below).

Pad the wrist or foot.

Slip the restraint knot over the padding.

Tighten until secure but not binding. (You should be able to slip two fingers inside the restraint.)

Tie the restraint ends to the frame of the bed, with a square knot.

There are many kinds of restraints in use. Here are some:

a length of quilted material

a length of heavy muslin

a length of heavy cotton tape with attached foam plastic and self-fastening cuff

mitt restraints

REMEMBER: Never use gauze or ropes to restrain a patient. They cut the skin and interfere with circulation.

Many commercial styles of restraints are available and often used. These have the advantages of allowing greater patient comfort and being easier to apply. Some types are disposable. Before applying, read package instructions carefully and then follow them exactly.

Making Knots

A Restraint Knot

Place one end of the material on a flat surface while you hold the other.

Make a figure eight next to the end of the flat surface.

Thread the end you hold through the two loops of the figure eight, keeping the other end free.

Adjust the loop to fit the ankle or wrist.

Knot once to fasten.

Tie the ends to the bed with a square knot.

A Square Knot

Hold an end in each hand.

Place the right end over the left end and tie. Then place the left end over the right end and tie.

Making an Unoccupied Bed

Equipment
  a mattress cover
  a pillow
  a pillowcase
  two full sheets
  a cotton drawsheet
  a plastic drawsheet
  a blanket
  a spread

Remove all bedding.

Fold the bottom sheet in half lengthwise.

Lay the lengthwise fold along the center of the mattress.

Pull the sheet toward the head until the foot edge reaches just to the mattress edge.

Open the sheet.

Tuck in the top of the sheet on the side where you stand.

Make a square corner at the top.

Tuck in the side of the sheet, working from the top to the bottom.

Lay the folded plastic sheet across the middle of the bed with the fold at the center.

Open the plastic sheet.

Place the cotton drawsheet on top of the plastic sheet and in the same way.

Be sure all the plastic is covered by the cotton sheet.

Tuck in both the plastic and cotton sheets together.

Go to the other side of the bed.

Tuck in the head of the bottom sheet and make a square corner.

Smooth the plastic and cotton drawsheets. Tuck them in together in three tight tucks: middle, top, bottom.

Return to the other side of the bed.

Fold the top sheet lengthwise and lay the fold along bed center so that the top of the sheet is just to the head edge of the mattress. Open the lengthwise fold.

Lay the lengthwise folded blanket so that the top edge of the blanket is 6 inches below the top edge of the sheet. Open the blanket.

Smooth and tuck the sheet and blanket together under the foot of the mattress.

Make a square corner and tuck once.

Lay the lengthwise folded spread on the bed so that the top edge of the spread reaches to the head edge of the mattress. Open the spread. Cuff the top of the spread under the blanket, then cuff the sheet top over that.

Smooth and tuck the spread under at the foot.

Make a square corner but do not tuck under the last flap; the spread side hangs free.

Go to the other side.

Complete that side in the same manner.

Return to the chair side.

Put on the pillowcase and place the pillow on the bed with the open pillowcase end facing the bedside stand.

Making an Occupied Bed

Close the door to the patient's room.

Tell him what you are going to do.

Lower the bed rests until the mattress is flat.

Remove the spread and the blanket. Leave the top sheet in place. Very often a bed is made just after the patient has had a bed bath. When this is the case, the cotton blanket is left on the patient while the bottom of the bed is being made. Then the clean top sheet is exchanged for the cotton blanket.

Have the patient help you pull up the mattress by positioning him flat on his back with knees flexed, soles against the mattress, and arms raised overhead so that he can grasp the head of the bed. Pull together on a count of three.

Ask the patient to turn on his side with his back to you. If the patient is helpless, go to the other side of the bed, turn the patient to you, and raise the side rail. Then return to the chair side of the bed. The side rail permits you to move the patient safely to the edge of the bed.

Pull the cotton drawsheet, the plastic sheet, and the bottom sheet free from under the mattress.

Roll the cotton drawsheet tight against the patient's back.

Lift the plastic sheet over the patient's back.

Roll the bottom sheet tight against the patient's back, exposing the mattress.

Fold a clean sheet lengthwise and lay the fold on the bed as close to the patient's back and the center of the bed as possible.

See that the foot of the sheet reaches just to the mattress edge.

Open the sheet and roll the top half tight against the patient's back.

Tuck the head of the sheet under the mattress and make a square corner.

Tuck the side of the sheet under the mattress, working from the head to the foot.

Lift the plastic sheet back over the rolled-under sheet and into place.

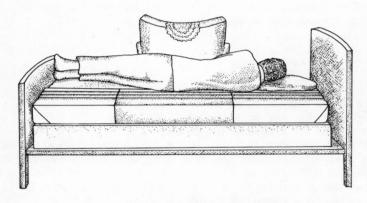

*Making an occupied bed. Note: Chair is
used as rail to protect patient from falling.*

Tuck it under the mattress.

Fold a clean drawsheet in half and lay it on the plastic sheet with the fold close to the patient.

Open the drawsheet and roll the top half tight against the patient's back.

Tuck the bottom half under the mattress.

Turn the patient to you, rolling him over the linen pushed against his back. Raise the side rail if necessary. Go to the other side of the bed.

Lower the side rail if in use.

Pull the soiled bedding free from the mattress.

Remove the soiled bottom sheet. Pull the clean sheet from under the patient and into place.

Tuck the bottom sheet under the head of the mattress.

Pull the side tight and make a square corner.

Tuck that side, working from the head to the foot and pulling the sheet smooth under the patient.

Pull the plastic sheet tight and tuck it in.

Pull the drawsheet tight and tuck it in.

Turn the patient on his back.

Return to the chair side of the bed.

Remove the pillow from under the patient's head.

Take off the soiled case and put on a clean one.

Replace the pillow under the patient's head.

Lay the clean top sheet over the soiled top sheet.

Remove the soiled sheet from under the clean top sheet.

Adjust the top sheet so that the sides hang evenly and there is enough material for a 6-inch cuff under the patient's chin.

Place the blanket over the top sheet.

Make a pleat, for foot space, in the center foot of the blanket and sheet. Tuck these together under the mattress. This prevents pressure on the patient's feet. Such pressure can cause foot drop, or permanent damage to the foot.

Make a square corner and tuck the side in once.

Put on the spread.

Tuck under the foot (no pleat).

Make a square corner, but do not tuck in the side.

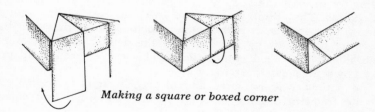

Making a square or boxed corner

9

Bathing, Skin Care, Massage, and Grooming

Bathing

In a recent study of the healing methods used by ten different cultures, among which were American medical practice, Navajo healing ceremonies, and Chinese folk medical practice, bathing was found to be an important aspect of treatment and healing in all of the cultures. Bathing not only cleanses the body but has positive subconscious meaning to a patient.

Many doctors think that a daily tub bath or shower is not good for some patients. They believe that daily bathing is too tiring, too drying for the skin, and exposes the patient to unnecessary chilling and falling. They think that once or twice a week is often enough for certain patients to bathe. Other doctors claim that any bad effects of daily bathing are less than the desirable effects of the general activity, blood stimulation, and sense of well-being produced by being clean and cared for.

The patient who is active and physically fit is better able to tolerate frequent bathing than one with a condition that causes unusual pain.

The patient with a short-term illness, such as a cold, may need to discontinue tub or shower bathing during the illness.

The patient who has no control of his bladder or bowel function certainly needs a bath more frequently than a patient who has good body control.

The patient's wishes also play a large part in the plan for his care. It is cruel to needlessly deny this pleasure to a person who throughout his lifetime enjoyed a daily bath. It is equally cruel to insist that a person must bathe whether or not he needs or likes it.

The time for a bath should also be flexible. Some patients like to bathe in the evening, others in the afternoon or as soon as they awaken in the morning. Whenever possible, allowances should be made for such preferences.

Regardless of how often a full bath is given to a patient, certain parts of the body should get washing and other skin care once or several times daily. These are the

face
hands
underarms
genitals
feet
bony parts (elbows, knees, spine)

Morning Care

On awakening, most people feel the need to urinate, clean their mouth, wash their face and hands, comb their hair, and dress before breakfast. Patients have these wants too, but they may require more time and more help to accomplish them than does the average adult.

Some patients are often stiff when they awaken, and movement may be slow and painful. Time must be allowed for this, and patience is necessary. Patients dislike being rushed, and if pushed, may resist instead of cooperating.

Old people are sometimes confused on awakening and need to be oriented. The way you greet them can mean the difference between relative independence and total dependence.

Your greeting should establish in the patient's mind who he is, who you are, where you are, what time it is, what you are going to do, and what is expected of him. Speak in a cheerful voice that is clear and distinct. Speak in short sentences.

Levels of Morning Care

Morning care for some patients may be no more than an awakening greeting. Others may need much more help.

To urinate, a patient may require
    help in walking to the bathroom;

help in using a commode;
a bedpan or urinal;
care for incontinence.

To give mouth care a patient may require
a reminder to brush his teeth;
preparation of mouthwash and toothbrush;
preparation of activities of daily living (ADL) equipment for
tooth care;
your brushing of his teeth;
special mouth care for a very ill or unconscious patient.

To wash his face and hands a patient may require
a reminder to do so in the bathroom;
preparation of water and washcloth in the bathroom;
preparation of ADL aids;
a basin of water, a washcloth, soap, and a towel at his bedside;
your washing of his face.

To comb his hair, the patient may require
a reminder to do so;
preparation of comb, mirror, and other equipment;
preparation of ADL equipment;
partial help with combing;
complete combing by you.

To dress, the patient may require
no help;
a reminder to do so;
some help;
preparation of ADL aids;
total help.

Evening Care

This care should be given to all patients at night before they
retire. It should be given to all bed patients in the late afternoon
as well as at night.

Equipment
the same as for morning care
a clean gown
a clean drawsheet

Offer a bedpan or urinal.

Bathe the patient's face and hands.

Give mouth care.

Wash the patient's back.

Rub the patient's back with lotion.

Straighten the bed clothing. Put a clean drawsheet on the bed, if needed.

Change the patient's gown.

Check to see that his water glass and tissues are within his reach and that his bell and light switch are at hand.

Position the bed as flat as allowed.

Remove extra pillows, if desired.

Put an extra blanket on the bed, if needed.

Provide air and a lower room temperature.

Put out the light, if desired.

Washing the Patient's Face and Hands

Equipment
   a basin of warm water
   a washcloth
   a face towel
   soap in a dish

Follow the general rules for any treatments when the patient is able to care for himself.

Position him and place the equipment so that he can wash himself. If the patient cannot wash himself, you must bathe him.

Dip the cloth in the clean water.

Wring it well and make a mitt to cover your hand.

Wipe the patient's eyes, starting at the nose and wiping outward. Then wipe the rest of the face.

Do not use soap on the face unless the patient wants it.

Put the towel on the bed by the patient's near hand.

Put the basin on the towel.

Place both of the patient's hands in the basin.

Do not put the cake of soap into the water.

Soap your own hands and use them to soap the patient's.

Use the washcloth to rinse the hands.

Remove the basin.

Wipe the patient's hands on the towel.

Bathing Your Patient

It is important to keep the skin of any patient in good condition because the skin helps rid the body of waste. Perspiration brings wastes to the skin surface. Bathing the skin removes the wastes and helps keep pores unplugged. Bathing gives a mild form of exercise and generally stimulates body functions. Bathing also makes a patient feel more comfortable, refreshed, and cared about. A daily bath or other skin care (usually both) is given to every

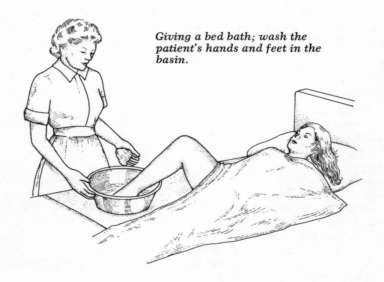

Giving a bed bath; wash the patient's hands and feet in the basin.

patient. Any signs of redness, rash, or pressure must be reported to the doctor.

A COMPLETE BED BATH

A bed bath is given when the doctor orders complete bed rest for the patient, or when the patient is unable to bathe himself.

It is best to follow the same order or procedure each time a complete bed bath is given. This order is as follows: eyes, face, neck, ears, chest and abdomen, far arm, near arm, hands, far leg, near leg, feet, back, buttocks, genitals.

This order of procedure is designed to use the cleanest water on areas where that is desirable, and to standardize the steps so that you always know which part of the body has been washed and which has not.

Bath water for a bed bath should be changed before the back, buttocks, and genitals are washed.

Prevent chilling the patient by working as quickly as possible, by keeping all of the patient covered except for the part that you are bathing, and by drying the skin thoroughly.

Use soap with caution. Overuse can make rinsing difficult and an irritating residue may be left on the patient's skin.

Bathtime offers a natural time to talk with and observe the patient. You should be alert for anything that might contribute to the diagnosis and treatment of the patient.

Equipment
    a bath towel
    a face towel
    a washcloth
    a cotton blanket
    clean bed linen (if the bed is to be made)
    a toothbrush
    toothpaste
    a glass of mouthwash or dentifrice
    an emesis basin
    a comb and brush
    a hair tonic or cream
    soap in a dish
    alcohol or skin lotion and bath powder (The choice of alcohol or lotion would depend on the patient's skin. Alcohol would be used on oily skin, lotion on dry.)
    a large basin of water at 110° F. (43° C.). Test it with a bath thermometer. (This is the ideal temperature to prevent chilling or burning the patient. Bring the water last so it won't cool through waiting.)
    a nail brush, scissors, nail file or emery board, hand lotion

Follow the general rules for all treatments.

Lower the bed if elevated and if lowering is allowed.

Remove unneeded pillows. One can be left under the head if the patient desires.

Put the cotton blanket over the patient as you fanfold the top covers to the foot of the bed. Be sure the feet are free.

Face, Neck, and Ears. Remove the patient's gown.

Lift the patient's head and spread the large towel across his pillow.

Spread the face towel under his chin.

Wet the washcloth and wring it so it does not drip.

Make a bath mitt of the cloth by wrapping it around your palm and fingers, holding it with your thumb. Tuck the edges under so they don't drag.

Wash the eyes gently, from the nose outward, with plain water. Use a separate corner of the washcloth for each eye.

Wash the face, forehead, nose, and cheeks with plain water. (Use soap only if necessary.)

Rinse in the same way.

Do not put the soap into the bath water at any time.

Wrap a corner of the face towel around your hand to prevent its dragging and dry the face.

Wash the neck and ears in the same way. Wash the far ear first, then the neck, then the near ear.

Rinse and dry.

Chest and Abdomen. Remove the towel from under the patient's head and spread it across his chest.

Pull the cotton blanket and other towel down to the abdomen.

Soap, rinse, and dry the chest and sides of the chest, working under the towel. Pay special attention to the area under the breasts.

Powder under the breasts if they are heavy.

Leave the towel over the chest. Pull the cotton blanket lower to expose the entire abdomen.

Soap, rinse, and dry the abdomen, the sides of the abdomen, the upper part of the hips, and the front pubic area. Use long, smooth strokes to avoid pressure and tickling.

Pull up the blanket and remove the towels.

Arms and Hands. Bring the far arm and shoulder across the patient's chest.

Place the large towel under the arm.

Soap, rinse, dry, and observe the arm, including the axilla (armpit).

Remove the towel and place it under the near arm.

Soap, rinse, and dry the arm, including the axilla.

Remove the towel and spread it on the bed under the patient's near hand.

Put the basin on the towel and have the patient put both hands into the water.

Soap your hands and use them to soap the patient's hands. Use a nailbrush, if needed.

Rinse. Remove the basin. Dry the hands thoroughly. Put hand lotion on, if desired. Observe the hands and give nail care as needed.

Legs and Feet. Arrange the cotton blanket to expose the far leg and cover the rest of the body.

Have the patient flex (bend) the far knee.

Spread the towel under the leg.

Soap, rinse, dry, and observe the leg.

Repeat the procedure with the near leg.

Flex both knees.

Place the towel on the bed between the feet. Place the basin on the towel.

Lift the feet into the basin and allow them to soak. If the feet are large or the patient helpless, bathe one foot at a time in the basin.

Soap with your hands. Use the nailbrush, if needed. Rinse. Remove the basin and place the feet on the towel.

Dry well between the toes. Observe and give nail care as needed.

Apply lotion or powder. Remove towel.

Back and Buttocks (or Hips). Help the patient turn onto his far side. Adjust his position so that he is comfortable and you can work easily.

Change the bath water.

Uncover the patient's back.

Spread the large towel under his back and buttocks. Soap, rinse, dry, and observe the patient's neck, back, and buttocks. Use long, firm strokes.

Rub the patient's back, giving special attention to pressure areas (shoulders and hips). Use hand or body lotion or alcohol. Then powder. SEE: Skin Care, Massage.

Replace the patient onto his back.

Genitalia. Put a towel under the patient's buttocks.

Place the bath basin, soap, and towel within the patient's reach and, if he is able, allow him to wash, rinse, and dry himself.

If he is unable, you must do it for him.

It is easiest to wash a patient's genitals by placing him on a bedpan. Then use a pitcher to pour some warm water over the genitals. Use the cloth mitt to soap the genitals. Pour more water to rinse. Dry well. The towel and cloth used to bathe the genitals should not be reused until laundered.

AFTER A BATH

Give mouth care (see page 126). (This may be done before the bath if desired.)

Spread a towel under the patient's head.

Comb and arrange his hair.

Allow the patient to use deodorant, cologne, or makeup, if desired.

Help the patient into a clean gown.

Make the bed with clean linen.

Clean and put away equipment.

Report any unusual condition observed during the bath.

GIVING A PARTIAL BED BATH

You need the same equipment as for a bed bath.

Position the patient comfortably.

Place all the equipment within his reach.

Allow him to bathe all of himself but his back and feet.

Wash his feet and back in the same ways as for a bed bath.

Allow him to wash his genitals.

Apply skin lotion to his entire body.

AFTER A BATH

Give mouth care. (This may be done before the bath if desired.)

Spread a towel under the patient's head.

Help him to comb and arrange his hair.

Allow the patient to use deodorant, cologne, or makeup, if desired.

Help the patient into a clean gown.

Make the bed with clean linen.

Clean and put away equipment.

GIVING SHOWERS AND BATHS

See that the bathroom is clean, warm, and draft-free.

Help lay out the patient's clean clothes in his room.

See that the patient's room is warm and draft-free.

See that special equipment (eyeglasses, hearing aids) are safely stored.

See that the patient has with him any necessary adaptive equipment (soap on string, long-handled brush).

Take the patient to the bathroom in a wheelchair if possible.

If a shower bench or regular chair is to be used, place it in the shower stall before the patient enters.

A shower chair is a small-sized straight chair on wheels. On some, the chair seat is cut out for easier bathing of the genitals. Some types can be used as bath, commode, and shower chairs. The wheels on the chair can be locked. SEE: Wheelchairs.

Turn on and test the strength, direction, and temperature of the shower spray *before the patient enters*. Adjust the spray to a gentle one, aimed to reach the patient below shoulder level. The temperature should be warm (110° F.; 43° C.) — never hot. Fill the tub and test the water temperature before the patient enters.

Unless a shampoo is intended, see that the patient wears a shower cap.

Remove a condom urinary drainage set if the patient is wearing one.

Be sure brakes are locked on a shower chair while it is in the stall.

Even when the patient is able to bathe himself, if he is weak do not leave him alone in the bathroom.

Help the patient to wash himself, as needed, but allow him to do as much as possible for himself.

Do not allow him to stay longer than necessary in the shower or bath.

Do not expose the patient's nude body unnecessarily.

Wear a plastic apron to protect yourself.

For the aged patient, a shower is often the preferred means of bathing. It is easier and safer than transferring in and out of a tub. It takes less time and causes less strain on a patient. A shower chair can be rolled into the shower and allows the patient greater security and comfort.

HELPING WITH A BATH OR SHOWER

A tub bath or shower is given when the doctor orders OOB ("out of bed") or ambulatory ("can walk about") for the patient's activity. Sometimes the doctor orders BRP, which means "bathroom privileges." He may order *shower only* or *tub bath*.

Equipment
    a nonskid floor mat
    a washcloth, soap, and towels
    body lotion or powder
    a change of clothing
    for a bath: *a rubber suction bathtub mat; a bathtub seat or stool with safety tips on the legs*
    for a shower: *a plastic apron; a shower cap*

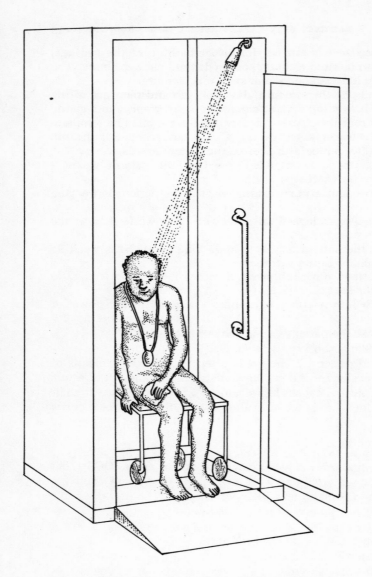

Using a shower chair and shower safety holds.
Note: Ramp to admit small wheelchair backed into
shower. Gentle shower spray hits patient's shoulders
but not his head. Soap is on a string around
patient's neck.

Dress the patient in robe and slippers but leave him in a comfortable place in his room.

Gather all necessary equipment.

Prepare the bathroom. Be sure that both tub and room are clean and no water is on the floor. Warm the room to 75° F. (23° C.) or more. Be sure that there are no drafts. Run the water to fill a third of the tub. Test the water temperature. It should be comfortably warm (110° F; 43° C.). This is the best temperature — it cannot burn or chill.

Return to the bedroom. See that it is warm and draft-free.

Help the patient to the bathroom.

Have him sit on the chair to remove his clothing. Place his clothing where it cannot get wet.

If a patient is modest and does not want to bare his genitals, tie a gauze strip around his waist. Loop a small towel through the strip so that it covers the genitals.

Tub Bath. Help the patient onto the side of the tub, then into the tub and onto the seat.

Let him bathe himself as much as possible.

Wash his back for him. If the patient sits high in the tub, use a pot to pour water over his body.

Bathe him quickly. Do not let him stay in the tub for a long time.

Never turn on or let the patient turn on the hot water tap while he is in the bathtub. There is danger of accidental burns from the water being too hot. Add additional hot water by drawing it from the sink tap into a pan. Test the water temperature before adding it to the bath water.

Dry the top of the patient's body while he is still in the tub.

Grasp him under the armpits to help him out of the tub.

Apply body lotion, powder, etc., as desired.

Help the patient dress.

Help him back to his room, and either to bed or to a comfortable place where he can rest.

Shower. The procedure for a shower is much the same.

Place one chair or stool in the shower and one outside the shower.

Wear a plastic apron to avoid wetting yourself.

Adjust the spray before the patient enters. Test the temperature. Do not have the spray forceful or positioned so that it could strike the patient's face.

Place the soap and washcloth within the patient's easy reach.

Unless you plan to wash the patient's hair, have him wear a shower cap.

Do not leave a patient alone in the tub or shower if he is weak or

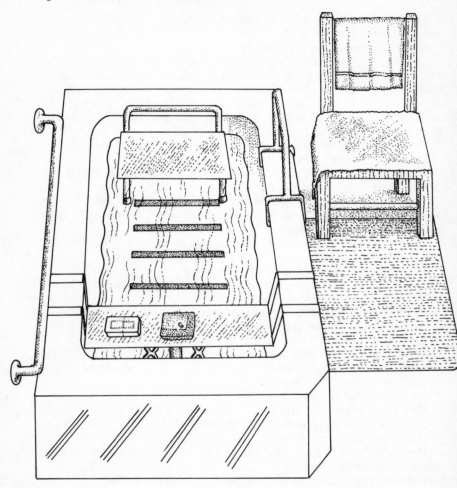

*A tub ready for a patient's bath. Note: Tub tray with soap
and washcloth. Safety strips on tub bottom. Strong stool in
bathtub. Water already drawn in bathtub. Safety hand-
holds on tubside and far wall. Suction mat at tubside. Straight
chair at tubside, seat covered with a towel. Other folded towel
at back.*

has any mental confusion. A patient is considered to be confused if his actions or speech are in any way abnormal, or if he is under certain medications, alcohol, or drugs.

At home, you can improvise a wheelchair to get a heavy patient to a tub by attaching roller casters to the four legs of a strong straight chair. This makes an easy chair to roll through narrow doorways.

Footbath

A footbath allows a patient to soak and clean his feet without wetting the rest of his body.

Equipment
    a comfortable chair
    a plastic sheet
    a bathmat or towel
    a towel
    a washcloth
    a basin large enough to hold the patient's feet
    enough water at 100° F. (40° C.) to fill the basin a third full
    soap
    skin lotion and powder

Help the patient to remove his shoes and stockings or socks. See that his pants are rolled up or removed.
Place the plastic sheet under the patient's feet.
Place the bathmat over the plastic sheet.
Fill the basin a third full and place on the mat near the patient's feet.
Help the patient to place his feet in the water.
Help the patient, as needed, to wash his feet.
Remove his feet from the basin.
Help him to dry them thoroughly.
Inspect the condition of the feet.
Give nail care if needed.
Apply lotion and powder.
Help the patient to get dressed.
Clean and put away all equipment.

Genital Bath or Perineal Care

The patient with urinary dribbling or rectal or vaginal leaking requires frequent daily genital and rectal washing. Here is a simple and quick way to bathe the genital area.

Equipment
    a large pitcher of warm (100° F.; 40° C.) soapy water
    a large pitcher of warm (100° F.; 40° C.) clear water
    two disposable washcloths
    a plastic disposable bag
    skin lotion
    a clean genital pad or dressing

Remove soiled genital pad. Put it in the plastic disposable bag.
Seat the patient on the toilet, commode, or bedpan.
Pour the soapy water slowly over the genital and rectal area.
Use one washcloth to clean off any soil. Wipe in one direction only, from front to back.
Discard washcloth into disposable bag.
Pour clear water over the genital and rectal area.
Pat dry with second washcloth. Dry from front to back.
Discard washcloth into disposable bag.
Help patient off the toilet, commode, or bedpan.
Apply skin lotion.
Put on clean genital pad or dressing.

Sitz Bath

A sitz bath allows a patient to soak his buttocks and genitals without wetting the rest of his body.

Equipment
    a strong, straight, low chair
    a plastic sheet
    two towels
    a washcloth
    a small basin large enough for the patient's buttocks
    enough water at 100° F. (40° C.) to fill the basin a third full
    soap
    skin lotion and powder

Drape the plastic sheet over the chair seat.

Cover the plastic sheet with a folded towel.

Fill the basin a third full of water.

Place the basin on the chair.

Help the patient remove his lower clothing. (Socks and stockings may be left on.) Roll stockings below knees.

Help him to sit in the basin.

Help him to wash himself, if necessary.

Help him to stand and dry himself.

Inspect the genitals and buttocks for redness or irritation.

Help the patient to apply lotion and powder.

Help him get dressed.

Remove and clean equipment.

Skin Care

A patient's skin can reveal many things about his life. It can show his parentage, the climate in which he lived, his diet, how active he has been, how long he has lived, and how filled with emotions, illnesses, and injuries his life has been. Through the years, these factors change a person's skin so that it looks different from the time of his youth.

With age the skin loses strength, elasticity, and the ability to hold moisture and heal. It becomes folded, lined, wrinkled, lax, dry, cracked, calloused, flabby, crusty, and scarred. Dark spots, broken blood vessels, moles, and other growths appear. Head and body hair thins and grays, while ear, nose, and facial hair increases. The skin becomes less resistant to irritation, infection, injury, bruising, allergic reactions, and breakdown.

It is easy to see, then, that good skin care is a necessity for every patient. Since every patient is different, however, a skin care plan should be the one best suited to the individual patient's needs.

Any plan for good skin care of a patient must include all of the following:

a good diet
enough fluid intake
good bowel and urinary function
physical activity
inspection of the skin
bathing of the skin

hair care
care of the feet and nails
massaging and oiling of the skin
proper bedding and clothing
proper body alignment

Diet, Fluid Intake, and Bowel and Urinary Function

Encourage, oversee, prepare, and help the patient in the best possible ways to eat the diet and drink the fluids that are right for him. Encourage, oversee, prepare, and help the patient to eliminate his body wastes in the manner best for him.

Physical Activity

It is your duty to encourage, oversee, prepare, and help the patient to move and change position in the best possible ways for him. This means that you must offer him regular reminders to walk, stand, use adaptive equipment, and perform activities of daily living, occupation, and recreation if he is capable of these things. To a helpless bed patient, it may mean your faithful turning of him every two hours.

Inspection of the Skin

WHEN TO INSPECT

Inspection is a very important aspect of skin care because the skin of an ill person loses sensitivity, and a patient may not feel discomfort or pain until a condition has become severe. The skin of any patient should be inspected at every opportunity. These include

during morning and afternoon care;
during bathtime;
during bowel and urinary care;
during dressing and undressing;
before and after use of adaptive equipment;
during back care;
during changing of incontinent patients;
during turning of bed patients;
during treatments;
on the complaint of any patient about itching, burning, soreness, numbness, or other changes in any part of the skin.

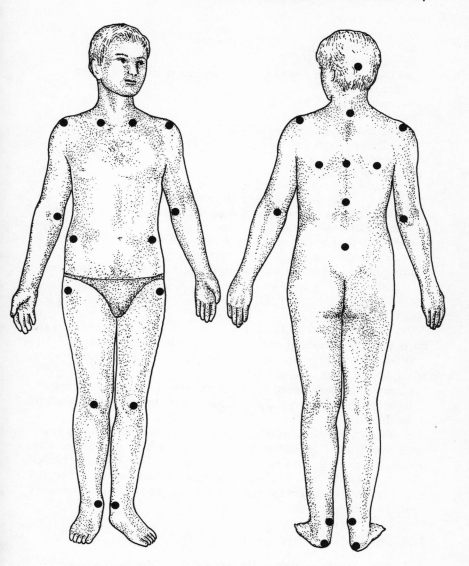

Body front and back areas most sensitive to skin breakdown.

WHERE TO INSPECT
  the scalp
  the hairline
  behind the ears
  the face and neck (especially around the mouth and eyes)
  under the arms
  the hands (front, back, and nails)
  under the breasts
  inside any large folds or fat rolls
  the elbows (front and back)
  the genitals and anus
  the shins and calves
  the knees (front and back)
  the feet (soles, heels, between the toes, nails)
  the entire back (especially the shoulder blades, spinal ridge, and buttocks)
  any area that is pressured by a piece of adaptive equipment, a cast, or clothing
  any area that has been injured, bruised, or shows redness or rash

WHAT TO LOOK FOR

Texture changes: unusual smoothness, roughness, scaling, goose flesh, graining, crusting, welts, rashes, chafing, and irritation.

Color changes: redness, blueness, graying, blackening, white spots, brown spots, and so forth.

Growths: moles, warts, tumors, callouses, corns, and so forth.

Injuries: bruises, scratches, scrapes, cuts, burns, infections, and so forth.

Pressure sores or decubitus ulcers: a very red, sometimes blackened, open sore, appearing on the body where unusual pressure occurs. This can be over any bony part, such as the shoulder blades, elbows, along the spinal ridge, or heels. It can also occur under very heavy breasts or other fat rolls and on areas rubbed by adaptive equipment or casts.

Proper Bedding and Clothing

A firm mattress allows for better distribution of a patient's weight and therefore prevents unusual pressure on any one part of the body. It also allows for easier turning and positioning of the patient. Special mattresses that constantly redistribute body weight are available; these are helpful for the patient whose skin is nearing breakdown or has an existing bedsore.

Bedclothing should be kept clean, dry, and free of wrinkles. Moisture and wrinkles irritate the skin.

Soft, lightweight sheets, pillowcases, and bedcovers help prevent irritations.

Personal clothing should be loose, comfortable, soft, lightweight, and clean. Nothing that cuts off blood circulation, such as garters or elastic girdles, should be worn. Both bedclothing and personal clothing should be laundered in mild, nonirritating soap or detergent.

Proper Body Alignment

Position the patient, whether standing, sitting, or in bed, so that his weight is evenly distributed and there is no interference with blood supply. This is very important in maintaining skin health.

Care of a Patient Threatened by Skin Breakdown and Bedsores or Decubitus Ulcers

Special care should be started at the first sign of redness or breakdown of the skin. The area should be brought to the attention of the doctor. Measures should be taken to stop the pressure on the immediate area and to encourage healing. These procedures vary from one doctor to another, but they may include

increased physical activity and repositioning to relieve pressure on the sensitive area;

a special mattress to redistribute weight constantly;

a sheepskin under the back to cushion and redistribute weight and increase blood supply to the area. The sheepskin is placed so that the wool is next to the patient's skin. The sheepskin may be real or synthetic. It is soft, easily washed and dried, and generally well tolerated by the patient;

self-adhering foam padding on pressure points (rubber rings or doughnuts are not recommended because they tend to cause other pressure points);

heel protectors;

normal saline solution to wash an ulcer;

medication for the area (on doctor's orders);

a hair dryer set on cool or other means to dry and stimulate
blood circulation to an ulcer (on doctor's orders);

increased massaging and oiling of the surrounding area;

for an incontinent patient, a urinary catheter or condom drainage (on doctor's orders);

a cut-out seatboard for a wheelchair patient (on doctor's
orders).

Regular Bathing of the Skin and Hair Care

See that the patient gets the regular bathing and shampooing
that is best suited to his particular needs. This may mean a weekly
bath and beauty shop appointment for the active patient with very
dry skin. To the incontinent patient it may mean back bathing
several times a day and a bed shampoo. Special mild soaps,
shampoos, and creams should be used.

Care of Feet and Nails

See that fingernails and toenails of a patient receive the specific
care needed by that individual. This can mean making appointments with a manicurist and a podiatrist or giving daily foot baths
to a patient prone to infection and arranging regular appointments
with his doctor to have his nails trimmed.

Massaging and Oiling of the Skin

Regardless of the individual bathing schedule of a patient, he
should receive a back massage and oiling of his skin as part of the
daily routine for morning and evening care and as often as needed.

Massage stimulates blood circulation and helps maintain skin
tone. Oiling prevents drying, cracking, flaking, and crusting. Both
make the patient feel and look better. Both help prevent his skin
from breaking down and decubitus ulcers from forming.

The face can be oiled with cleansing cream, moisturizing cream,
shaving cream, or aftershave cream lotion.

Hand lotion should be used after every washing.

Special lotions such as Lubriderm, baby lotion, and Vaseline
Intensive Care lotion are good for back care and body rubbing.
These do not leave oily surfaces but soak into the skin and make
it soft and pliable. Lotion should be applied at every opportunity;

this means at most inspection times. Inspection and oiling the skin should be included as steps in nearly all procedures of nursing care.

USING SELF-ADHERING FOAM PADDING
Available at drugstores.

Equipment
a basin with warm water
a disposable cloth or gauze sponges
foam padding
scissors

Clean the skin surrounding the area.
Cut out a piece of padding three or four times larger than the sore area.
Cut a hole in the padding to the size and shape of the sore area.
Remove the adhesive liner from the pad and put the pad over the area so that the sore part is framed by the padding.
Stick the padding to the skin.
If the patient is very heavy, several pads can be stacked to make a thicker covering around the area.

Massage

In recent years the use of massage in conjunction with other health care methods has increased. A comparative study of cultural healing methods revealed that in all cultures studied, touch and massage played important roles in health care.

Touching is the first language that an infant learns to interpret. The way that he learns it may control his feelings about others for all of his life. Adult touching has more than sexual meaning. It speaks of other things that are basic needs of all humans: acceptance, concern, tenderness. Massage effectively repeats this message to relax tense muscles and helps to clear them of toxic wastes in the form of lactic acid.

Three forms of massage are popular:

relaxation: superficial stroking
Swedish or therapeutic: deep muscle stimulation
Shiatsu: Japanese form of therapeutic massage and spine and

joint manipulation that also probes nerve centers by applying thumb pressure

Whether a massage is mostly relaxing or mostly stimulating
depends on which motions are mostly used, the amount of pressure
applied by the massager, the speed of the strokes, how many times
each stroke is repeated. The choice of these factors should depend
on the individual and the immediate situation. Obviously, a very
thin patient cannot tolerate the amount of pressure that a heavier
one can. Using massage techniques when applying skin lotion increases the absorption of oils into the skin.

Techniques

Effective massage techniques include these features.
Repeated long smooth strokes, done with the palms of both
hands, pressing strongly with the flow of blood circulation that is
returning to the heart and pressing lightly when the hands return
to their starting position.
Kneading or repeated gentle pinching of about three inches of
muscle and skin along a muscle in the direction of returning blood
circulation.
Using the edge of the hands in a repeated chopping movement.
Beginning a stroke with one hand while ending a stroke with the
other to produce an effect of three hands massaging.

Giving a Back Rub

Equipment
    lotion (to take the chill out of the liquid, place the bottle in a
        pan of warm water and let stand a few minutes)
    a bath towel

Position the patient on his far side or on his abdomen.
Expose the full back area.
Spread the towel under the patient's back and buttocks.
Apply the lotion to your hands.
Place both of your hands at the base of the spine with your
fingers pointing in the direction of the neck.
Rub upward on each side of the spine, applying pressure with
the palms of your hands and using long, smooth strokes to the
shoulders. Then use a series of circular motions to return your
hands to the base of the spine.

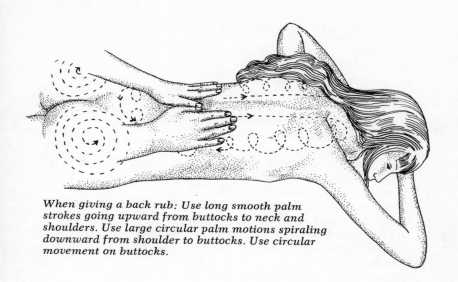

When giving a back rub: Use long smooth palm strokes going upward from buttocks to neck and shoulders. Use large circular palm motions spiraling downward from shoulder to buttocks. Use circular movement on buttocks.

Repeat several times, using more lotion as needed.
Massage the buttocks with large circular movements.
Then massage in circles inside of circles until all flesh has been rubbed.
Repeat several times.

Nail Care

When the services of a beauty parlor are available, many male and female patients choose to have their fingernails cared for by a beautician. The services of a podiatrist are usually available for older people, and this ensures good foot care. (Medicare sometimes pays for such services.) If these services are unavailable, however, you should give total nail care. You should always observe the nails at bathtime and correct immediate problems, such as broken nails or hangnails. A doctor or podiatrist should cut the toenails of a diabetic patient.

Equipment
    a plastic sheet
    a small washbasin half filled with water at 100° F. (40° C.)
    soap
    an orangewood stick

skin lotion
a soft nailbrush
nail scissors or clippers
an emery board

Position the patient comfortably near a table.
Cover the tabletop with plastic.
Fold the towel and put it over the plastic.
Bring a basin with water.
Help the patient to place hands in water.
Allow his hands to soak and wash.
Clean the nails well, using the orange stick and nailbrush.
Bring clean water to rinse hands and nails.
Dry hands and nails thoroughly.
Trim nails with clippers or scissors. Cut straight across, not around the nail.
Remove rough edges with emery board.
Apply skin lotion.

Hair Care

Any patient needs regular hair care: combing, washing, cutting, and setting. Groomed hair is not only necessary for personal cleanliness but it also gives a person a sense of well-being and is attractive to others. Because of these facts, many nursing facilities have beauty parlors and barber shops or arrange for these services to be brought to the patients on a regular basis. Whenever possible, this is the preferred means of washing, cutting, and setting hair.

When it is necessary or desirable to shampoo a patient's hair at home, consideration should be given to the patient's active strength and the patient's choice of methods before selecting from the following three:

shampoo in shower
shampoo at sink
shampoo in bed

Shampooing

See that the room is warm and draft-free.
Don't expose the patient's body more than necessary.

Protect the patient's clothing.

Handle the patient as gently as possible.

Brush hair before shampooing to help loosen dirt from scalp.

See that the patient's eyes are protected.

Plug ears with cotton to prevent water from running into them.

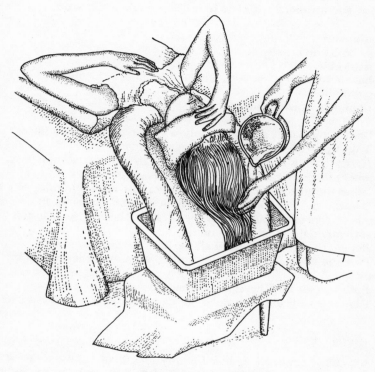

Washing a patient's hair in bed

Test water temperature before using. It should be **no** hotter than 105° F. (42° C.).

Use as little shampoo as possible.

Massage head with fingertips — never with nails.

A shampoo in the shower is best for any patient who can tolerate it.

Combing a Patient's Snarled Hair

Male patients seldom need help with their hair. If they do, combing and brushing is simple.

The longer hair of women can snarl and mat unless combed often and arranged with less hair at the back of the head.

Equipment
    a comb and brush
    a towel
    hair oil, a petroleum jelly such as Vaseline, or alcohol
    cotton balls
    ribbon or gauze bandage

Spread the towel across the pillow under the patient's head.

Take up a few strands of hair near the scalp.

If the hair is very tangled, apply hair oil, petroleum jelly, or alcohol to these strands with cotton balls.

Wind the strands about the first finger of your left hand.

Use the comb with your right hand. Comb the ends first. Then comb farther and farther up the strands, letting your left finger absorb any pulls from the comb.

Repeat the procedure until all the hair is combed.

Part the combed hair in the center and down the middle of the back.

Pull the hair to either side just behind the ears and braid.

Fasten each braid with ribbon or gauze bandage.

Washing a Patient's Hair in Bed

A patient confined to bed for any length of time will need an occasional shampoo. A bed shampoo should never be given without the permission of the doctor.

Equipment
    a low chair or stool
    two large pitchers of warm water (110° F.; 43° C.); the difference in temperature from that used in regular shampooing allows for cooling in the pitcher
    shampoo
    a pail
    a small plastic sheet

a large rubber or plastic sheet
a pillow in a plastic case
a washcloth
two bath towels
a cotton blanket
a face towel
a safety pin
a portable electric dryer (if possible)

Check the room for drafts and warmth.

Place the chair or stool at the bedside near the head.

Cover the chair or stool seat with the small plastic sheet.

Put the pail on the covered stool.

Lower the bed to a flat position.

Remove the pillow from under the patient's head.

Put the cotton blanket over the patient.

Position the patient on her back crosswise in the bed, with her head close to the edge of the bed where you stand.

Put the plastic-covered pillow under the patient's shoulders, so that the head is lower than the shoulders.

Place one bath towel around the patient's neck and pin it.

Roll three sides of the large plastic sheet to form barriers against the water.

Position the rolled plastic sheet under the patient's head so that the head is surrounded by the rolls and the ends fall over the bedside and into the pail.

Adjust the patient's head so that it hangs well within the rolled plastic sheet and slightly over the side of the bed.

Give the patient the washcloth to hold over her eyes.

Pour warm water over the patient's head until hair is wet. Pour gently to prevent splashing. Keep the flow away from the face.

Pour part of the shampoo onto the head, being careful not to apply any to the face.

Massage the scalp with both hands, using your fingertips but not your nails.

Rinse the hair well.

Apply shampoo again.

Rinse again.

Wring the patient's hair gently.

Dry the patient's forehead with the face towel and then wrap it around her hair to absorb some of the wetness.

Lift the patient's wrapped head and remove the rolled plastic. Place it in the pail.

Pull the pillow out from under the patient's shoulders and put it under her wrapped head.

Remove the face towel from the hair and replace it with a clean bath towel.

Squeeze the hair in the folds of the towel and gently rub the hair to dry.

When the towel is damp, unpin the towel from around the patient's neck, remove the damp head towel and replace it with the neck towel.

Continue rubbing and squeezing until most of the water is removed from the hair.

Use the hand dryer to finish the drying process.

Comb and set the patient's hair as desired.

Remove the plastic-covered pillow and replace with the usual pillow and case.

Report to the doctor anything unusual you observed during the shampoo.

Giving a Shampoo at a Sink

Equipment
   a portable shower hose
   a plastic sheet
   a small sponge pad
   two towels
   shampoo
   a washcloth
   cotton earplugs
   a hairbrush
   a portable electric dryer

Place the patient in a wheelchair or a straight chair, positioned close to and facing the sink.

Put the plastic sheet around the patient's neck and shoulders.

Put the towel over the plastic sheet.

Brush the patient's hair.

Attach the shower hose to the faucet; turn on and test water.

Lean the patient forward in the chair so that her head is over the sink.

Put the sponge pad under her chin.

Put the earplugs in her ears.

Give her the washcloth to hold over her eyes.

Wet the hair, apply shampoo, and massage scalp.
Rinse.
Apply shampoo again and rinse.
Turn off the water.
Wring the hair gently.
Sit the patient upright and remove eye pad and earplugs.
Bring the shoulder towel around her head. Dry hair.
Remove the plastic sheet.
Replace with the dry towel.
Remove the head towel and use dryer to dry hair.
Comb and set hair.
Remove and clean equipment.

Lice

A louse is a gray, wingless insect that attaches itself to the hairs of the head. Another variety, crab lice, live in the pubic hair and eyelashes. Lice live on human blood obtained through biting the skin. These bites cause itching. Scratching the bites can cause soreness and infection. Lice are not only an unpleasant nuisance, they can transmit diseases such as typhus. They can spread from person to person very rapidly. In 1973, sixty-nine schools on Long Island had to close because of infestation with head lice.

Signs of lice are: scratching, rash, complaints of itching, dandrufflike eggs or nits attached firmly to hairs.

The best care is prevention through frequent bathing, hairwashing, and clothes washing or cleaning. When infection does occur, obtain special shampoo containing one percent benzine hexachloride from any drugstore. This will kill the lice and nits. After shampooing, rinse the hair with a vinegar solution, which loosens eggs or nits. Comb with a fine comb (also obtained at any drugstore) to remove nits. Wash with disinfectant or dry clean any personal or bed clothing used by the infected person.

Shaving a Male Patient

Equipment
   a tray with: *a razor and blades; paper towels; a bowl of warm water; shaving cream or soap*
   two towels
   a basin of hot water
   aftershave lotion

Review the general rules for treatment. Follow those that apply.

Have a good light on the patient's face.

Have the patient sit erect, if allowed.

Spread one towel under his chin.

Dip the other towel in the basin of hot water.

Wring it as dry as possible.

Place it over the lower face and chin for several minutes. This softens the whiskers.

Put some shaving cream in the palms of your hands and rub your palms over the patient's face. This way you control the area covered with cream.

Use a paper towel to wipe your hands.

Stretch the patient's skin tight at all times. This prevents cutting the skin.

To shave, stroke upward in a long, smooth movement. Follow it with a similar stroke downward over the same area. This makes a close, neat shave, since all hairs do not grow in the same direction.

Position the patient's head as needed to help you.

Clean the razor on paper towels to remove hairs.

Dip the razor in the bowl of warm water to remove hairs.

Run steaming water over the face towel.

Wring it as dry as possible and spread it over the shaved area for several minutes.

Pat the face dry with the neck towel.

Apply shaving lotion to the palms of your hands and massage over the shaved area.

If you should cut the skin, use a styptic pencil to touch the spot. This stops the bleeding.

Tooth Care

Good tooth care prevents tartar, tooth decay, gum disease, and tooth loss. Tartar is hardened plaque, a sticky, colorless film of bacteria or germs that is constantly forming on the teeth and gumline. Plaque (pronounced *plak*) changes sugar into acid that can decay the hard outer surface of a tooth and attack the tooth's inner nerves and pulp. This causes tooth decay. Plaque also can cause gum infection. The first signs of this are swelling, tenderness, and bleeding of the gums. Unless the gum infection is treated at this early stage, the infection will progress so that the gums recede, the jawbone is affected, and teeth loosen and fall out. Most adult teeth are lost in this way.

Good tooth care consists of

a good diet;
careful daily cleansing;
regular checkups by a dental professional.

Good Diet

Proper eating contributes to oral health as well as to general health. Eating sweets can increase tooth decay. After eating anything, the bacteria on the teeth increase their activity for about twenty minutes. Between-meal snacks, particularly sweets, encourage the growth of plaque. Only eat sweets when you are able to rinse your mouth after eating. SEE: Feeding: Nutrition.

Cleaning

Thorough cleaning has two steps. The first step is flossing, or cleaning between the teeth with dental floss or dental tape. The second step is brushing.

Using Dental Floss

Obtain *unwaxed dental floss* from any drugstore.

Remove a length (about a foot) from the container.

Wrap thread ends around the first fingers of both hands to make a tight inch of thread between these fingers.

Start behind the last upper tooth on one side and move tooth by tooth to the last upper tooth on the other side and then proceed in the same manner to all of the lower teeth.

Work the thread gently up and down between the teeth, cleaning the side surfaces of each tooth and including the area below the gumline. Take care not to cut into the gum. Move your fingers to change the angle of the thread.

Use a clean section of the floss whenever a used part becomes soiled or frayed.

After flossing, rinse your mouth with clear water to wash away any debris dislodged by the cleaning.

Brushing

Equipment
a soft nylon brush with rounded ends on its bristles
toothpaste, tooth powder, or a mixture of salt and baking soda;
fluoride paste or powder also helps teeth to resist decay

Brush the inside of the front teeth with an up-and-down motion.
Brush the inside of the back teeth and the chewing surfaces with
short back-and-forth strokes.
Brush where your teeth meet your gums.

Visiting the Dentist

Finding a dentist is not difficult. Ask friends, relatives, your
doctor, the information service at a hospital, or a neighborhood
health center for the name of a good dentist.

A regular dentist or his specially trained assistant should check
your teeth every six months. The checking usually includes

a special cleaning;
examination for decay areas or gum disease;
X rays, if necessary.

The dentist may refer you to a dental specialist.

An *endodontist* only treats tooth pulp and tissues at the roots of
teeth.

An *oral surgeon* extracts teeth or does surgery on and around the
mouth.

An *orthodontist* applies braces and moves teeth to correct cracked
or badly spaced teeth.

A *pedodontist* treats only children.

A *periodontist* treats gum problems.

A *prosthodontist* makes and fits replacements for lost teeth or
parts of the mouth, jaw, and face.

Children's Teeth

A child should begin learning to brush his teeth at about age
two. Hold the brush with him as you clean his teeth.

The first dental visit should take place between the ages of two
and three.

The Patient's Own Teeth

Equipment
   a toothbrush
   toothpaste
   a glass of mouthwash or water
   a basin or plastic dish
   a face towel
   tissues
   a drinking straw, if desired

Follow the general rules for treatments.
Spread the face towel under the patient's chin.
Hold the toothbrush over the emesis basin and pour mouthwash or water onto the brush.
Apply a small amount of toothpaste to the brush.
If the patient is able to brush his teeth, hand him the brush.
Hold the basin under the patient's chin.
If he is unable to brush his teeth, insert the brush into his mouth and gently brush, using up-and-down strokes.
Let the patient rinse his mouth and spit into the basin.
Wipe his mouth with a tissue and then with the towel.

Dentures, or False Teeth

Equipment
   a toothbrush
   a solution of dentifrice (such as Kleenite or Polident) for
      dentures
   a gauze square or tissue

Clean dentures before giving other mouth care.
Remove a full denture by grasping it with a piece of gauze or tissue and tilting it away from the gum.
Remove a partial denture by lifting the metal clamp with your fingernail.
Soak dentures in the solution of dentifrice.
Take the dentures to the bathroom or utility room. Hold one denture at a time, in the palm of your hand, over a sink partly filled with water and brush under running water.
Place the dentures in a cup of clean water.
Return to the patient and place the dentures in a safe place.

Clean the patient's own teeth and allow him to rinse his mouth with mouthwash.

Special Mouth Care for the Helpless Patient

Equipment
a teaspoon with the handle wrapped with gauze bandage
a cup of mouthwash solution
a basin or plastic dish
tissues
a towel

Turn the patient's head to one side.
Spread the towel beneath his chin.
Dip the wrapped handle in mouthwash solution until it is wet but not dripping. Take the patient's cheeks on either side of the mouth between the thumb and fingers of one hand. Squeeze gently to open his mouth. Insert the handle between the patient's lips.
Swab the teeth, gums, and tongue with the wrapped handle.
Repeat as often as necessary to clean.
Change the gauze on the teaspoon handle if necessary.

This mouth care should be given every hour or so to unconscious or otherwise helpless patients.
A thin application of oil to the lips helps prevent cracking.
A coated tongue and foul breath are often part of illnesses that cause unconsciousness or helplessness. Also, the mouth of an unconscious or helpless patient tends to drop open, which causes the mouth to dry out. Frequent mouth care relieves these conditions and adds to the patient's comfort.

10

Toileting

Giving a Bedpan or Urinal

Equipment
    toilet paper
    a bedpan or a urinal
    a cover

Make a habit of holding a bedpan by its side instead of by the front. You cannot hold the pan by its front and avoid putting part of your hand inside of it.

Warm the bedpan by running hot tap water over the seat. It is sometimes difficult for a patient to void unless he is relaxed. Warming the pan makes it less shocking to him and helps him to relax.

Dry the pan.

Dust the pan seat with talcum powder. A dusting of talcum powder on a bedpan prevents the pan from sticking to a patient's skin.

Cover the pan or urinal with a clean, dry cloth.

Take the pan to the bedside.

Be sure the foot of the bed is not elevated. If the foot is elevated, urine is apt to run out of a pan or urinal.

Stand at the center of the bed on the patient's right side.

Hold the pan by its near side with your right hand.

Remove the pan cover and drape it over the back of the chair or on the footstead.

Position your patient. The best position is flat on his back with

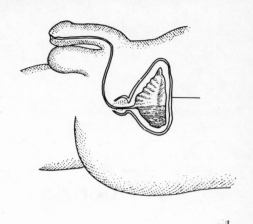

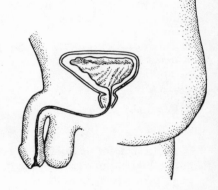

Urine does not completely empty from the bladder if a patient voids while lying down.

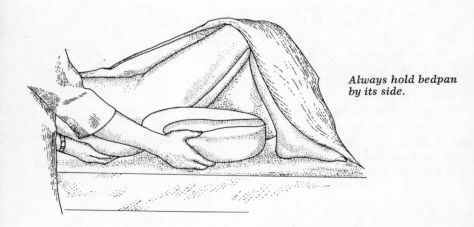

Always hold bedpan by its side.

the knees bent and the soles of his feet pressed flat against the mattress.

Position your left hand at the base of the patient's spine. Ask him to dig in his heels and lift his hips. As he does, you help lift his hips with your left hand and slide the pan into place with your right.

Raise the head of the bed, unless the doctor's orders forbid it. Raising the head of the bed often helps a patient to urinate or move his bowels because this is the normal position for these actions.

Put toilet paper within easy reach of the patient.

Be sure the signal bell is within the patient's easy reach.

When ready to remove the pan, reposition the patient flat on his back with his knees bent and the soles of his feet pressed against the mattress.

Remove the pan and put it on the chair seat. Cover with the bedpan cover.

Check the patient to be sure he is wiped clean.

If necessary, roll him to the far side and clean him.

Straighten the bedding.

Flush out and clean the bedpan and restore it to its place.

Make the patient comfortable.

When offering or receiving a urinal, remove the cover and hold the urinal by the bottom so that the patient can take the handle.

Giving a Bedpan to a Helpless Patient

Equipment
    toilet paper
    disposable moist tissue wipers or a basin of warm water and a
        cloth
    a bedpan
    a bedpan cover
    five pillows
    two sandbags with covers (two unopened two-pound coffee
        cans wrapped in towels can be used instead of sandbags)
    a cotton blanket
    a towel

Level the mattress.

Put the cotton blanket on the bed and fanfold the covers to the foot of the bed.

Go to the far side of the bed.

Raise the side rail or position a chair against the side of the bed.

Prop the pillows upright against the rail or chair back.

Return to the other side of the bed.

Move the patient close to the edge of the bed and turn him on his side toward you.

Place two of the pillows at his shoulder level. Cross the tops of these pillows so that they form an angle.

Center one pillow lengthwise beneath the crossed pillows in line with the length of the patient's spine.

Position the bedpan at the base of the lengthwise pillow so that it is aligned with the patient's buttocks.

Roll the patient back onto the pillows and bedpan.

Flex the patient's knees.

Fold the last pillow lengthwise, and slip the roll beneath the patient's knees.

Position the patient's feet together with soles flat against the mattress.

Place a sandbag on either side of the patient's feet.

To Remove the Pan

Remove the sandbags and the knee pillow.

Roll the patient toward you.

Clean the patient with toilet paper.

Wash the patient with moist tissue or warm water.

Dispose of papers into the bedpan unless fluid should be measured or a specimen obtained.

Remove the pan and place it on the bedside chair.

Remove the pillows.

Roll the patient onto his back.

Pull up the bedclothes and remove the cotton blanket.

A special smaller pan can be used for patients who are difficult to handle.

Sometimes a patient has a problem starting to urinate. The urge can be stimulated by the sound of running water. Turning on a faucet or pouring water from one glass to another is usually effective. Slowly pouring lukewarm water over the genitals while the patient is on the bedpan, commode, or toilet is also effective.

The Commode

A commode is an armed chair with an open seat that is higher than the one on a regular toilet. A removable container attaches beneath the commode seat. It is easier for a patient to transfer to a commode than to a toilet, and the commode gives better body support. The commode can be placed beside the bed or chair and the patient transferred directly onto it. After using the commode, the patient is wiped clean and returned to bed or chair. The commode container is removed, emptied, and cleaned in the same way as a bedpan. Disposable containers can be used on some commodes.

Toilet Grab Bars

These are waist-high, strong, bent, metal arms, placed on both sides of the toilet, so that the patient can support himself during

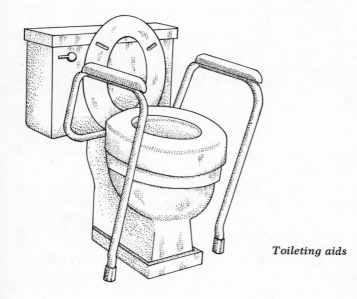

Toileting aids

the frequent insecurity of positioning himself on the toilet. Such bars make it possible for more ambulatory and wheelchair patients to use a regular toilet, although some may require your help in transferring to and from the toilet.

Bowel and Urine Control

Fecal Impaction

A stool that is allowed to remain in the lower bowel and rectum becomes hard and packed, and the patient finds it impossible to expel it.

When this occurs, the patient becomes ill. He may lose his appetite, experience nausea, vomit, have a fever, have chills, sweat, experience stomach cramps and other discomforts. His abdomen may swell and become hard. Sometimes he appears to have diarrhea, but it is only liquid seeping through the hard mass of impacted stool. There is only one thing to be done for this patient. The impacted feces must be removed by stimulation of the bowel with the index, or first, finger.

Some patients are susceptible to fecal impaction. If a patient's bowels do not respond well to the usual means of regulation ordered by the doctor (that is, diet, sufficient fluids, medications, enemas, and suppositories), then the doctor may remove the stool by digital stimulation. He usually orders a mineral oil enema or suppository to precede the digital stimulation by fifteen to twenty minutes.

The Incontinent Patient (one who has lost control of bowel or urinary function)

Common reactions of patients to incontinence are nervousness, disgust, anger, and depression. The patient may cry, moan, insist that he wants to die, scream, use abusive language, refuse to eat, demand constant attention, and refuse to cooperate or to take part in any activities.

Sometimes this kind of behavior seems exasperating and one may be tempted to ignore the patient, to avoid him as much as possible, to hurry through any necessary care, and to separate him from others who might be annoyed by him.

Nothing could be worse for the incontinent patient. Even if he is given the best physical care, such neglect and isolation are so psychologically harmful that they can destroy the patient's will to live.

Instead, this patient needs more attention. He needs understanding, respect, and affection. He needs to be reassured that

he is liked and accepted by others;
incontinence is not shameful;
incontinence can happen to anyone;
incontinence can be managed with a minimum of discomfort,
     embarrassment, and time;
an incontinent patient can lead a good, happy life.

Develop a plan of nursing care that meets both the physical and
the psychological needs of this patient. Such a plan might include

visiting with the patient at times when he doesn't need chang-
     ing or other nursing care;
including the patient in as many group activities as possible;
encouraging the patient to talk about his incontinence and
     how he can help with managing it;
instituting a toilet retraining program;
discussing the patient's interests during changing times;
organizing the changing process so that it is a quick, simple
     procedure;
giving special attention such as an extra dessert or a flower by
     the bedside; such attention, however, should be given freely
     and never as a reward for bowel and bladder control or
     cooperation.

CLEANING THE INCONTINENT BED PATIENT
Equipment
   a basin of warm water
   soap
   disposable washcloths
   disposable gloves
   bath towels
   newspaper or a large piece of disposable plastic
   a disposable bag
   toilet tissue
   clean sheets (as needed)
   disposable bedpads
   a clean gown
   air deodorizer

See that the room is warm and free of drafts.
Collect everything needed on the bedside table.
Draw the curtain around the patient's bed.
Level the mattress.

Tell the patient what you are going to do.

Remove the spread and blanket from the bed.

Spread the newspaper on the floor.

Loosen the top sheet.

Remove the patient's gown and put it on the newspaper.

Go to the far side of the bed.

Move the patient to the side of the bed that you are facing.

Turn the patient so that he faces you.

Raise the side rail on the bed.

Return to the other side of the bed.

Spread open the disposable bag (the bag can be placed into the patient's wastepaper container and the bag top cuffed over the top of the container).

Put on disposable gloves.

Turn back the top sheet to expose the patient's back, buttocks, and thighs.

Use toilet tissue to remove as much of the feces as possible from the patient's body and the sheets. Discard into the disposable bag.

Loosen the drawsheet and fold it so that a clean part is under the patient. Then roll the sheet against the patient's back.

Wet a disposable washcloth and remove the feces from the patient's body. Discard that cloth.

Use another washcloth to clean the patient thoroughly with soap and water. Rinse off all soap. Dry the patient.

Use the same washcloth and soap and water to clean the plastic drawsheet. Dry the sheet thoroughly.

Cover the roll of soiled drawsheet with a disposable bedpad.

Put a clean drawsheet (and bottom sheet, if needed) on that side of the bed.

Roll the patient to the clean side of the bed.

Raise the bedrail.

Go to the other side of the bed.

Lower the side rail.

Remove the soiled sheets from that side of the bed. Put them on the newspapers.

Wash and dry any part of the patient that is soiled.

Wash and dry any soiled part of the plastic sheet.

Make the bottom sheet on that side of the bed.

Rub the patient's back, buttocks, and thighs with skin lotion.

Notice any redness or rash.

Position the patient on his back.

Check the genitals to see that all areas are clean.

Return to the other side of the bed.

Lower the bedrail.
Change the disposable bedpad.

RETRAINING

A retraining program should be the outgrowth of an evaluation of the patient that includes an understanding of his specific physical, psychological, and social needs and capabilities. This knowledge should also determine the right moment for starting the program.

The program and procedure must be explained fully to the patient and to all nursing personnel and family members who will participate in it.

Regular progress reports and suggestions by the patient and nursing personnel are needed to sustain interest in the program.

Any program should include

an adequate diet;

frequent offerings of drinking water and other fluids;

the use of a sitting position regardless of whether the retraining is with a toilet, commode, or bedpan (bowel and bladder cannot empty completely when a patient is lying down);

discussion with the patient about his normal bowel and bladder habits and observation of his pattern of incontinence;

based on his habits and pattern, a daily twenty-four-hour schedule and record sheet that specifies the times for twenty minutes of toileting at every two-hour interval (once control is established, the schedule can be changed to every three or four hours);

the faithful carrying out of the schedule with no exceptions allowed;

the help and encouragement of nursing assistants during positioning and toileting;

a plan of physical exercise to stimulate and regulate bowel and bladder functions;

a plan of mental activity to distract the patient from thinking about himself;

use of items between toileting that prevent bed soiling, such as adult diapers, sanitary napkins, and shower caps filled with disposable tissues or gauze;

setting an alarm clock for the night schedule;

dressing the patient in street clothes during the day;

selecting street clothing that allows easy toileting.

Care of a Patient with Urinary Drainage

A doctor may order urinary drainage for a patient who is unable to control urinary flow. For female patients, and sometimes for males, the doctor orders indwelling catheter urinary drainage. For other males, the doctor orders condom urinary drainage.

FOLEY, OR INDWELLING, CATHETER DRAINAGE

The Foley catheter is a soft rubber catheter with a small inflatable balloon on the insertion tip. The catheter is inserted into the bladder under sterile conditions by a doctor or professional nurse. The balloon is then inflated. This prevents the catheter from slipping out of the bladder.

The catheter is attached to sterile, disposable, plastic tubing, and the end of the tubing is inserted into a sterile drainage bag. Several types of drainage bags are used. One type is attached to the side of the bed. Another type is fastened onto the patient's leg.

A Foley catheter can remain in a patient for several days.

Urinary Infection

Because an indwelling catheter irritates the membranes of the urethra and bladder, the patient is subject to urinary infection. Every effort to prevent such infection must be made through the careful attention of all nursing personnel. Every nursing care plan includes most of the precautions to be discussed here. Do not touch any part of an indwelling catheter drainage system unless you have been instructed in your specific duties by the doctor. If any part of a drainage system does not appear to be in correct position or working well, report to the visiting nurse or doctor at once.

Infections often start

around the catheter where it enters the body;
on the end of the drainage tube that is inserted into the drainage bag;
at the point where the catheter and drainage tube join.

PREVENTING URINARY INFECTION

Encourage the patient to drink plenty of fluids. Most patients with indwelling catheters are on measured intake and output and are expected to drink at least 3,000 cc. of fluid daily.

Prevent pull on the catheter by looping the drainage tube. Secure the loop to the bed by passing an elastic band around the tube and pinning the elastic to the drawsheet.

Watch the drainage tube and drainage bag to see that urine is flowing freely. Take special notice

when turning, dressing, or positioning a patient;
just after the catheter is attached to the drainage tube;
just after the catheter is inserted in the drainage tube.

Irrigate the bladder regularly with sterile solution. (This should always be done under the supervision of a professional nurse.) After bladder irrigation, flush the drainage tube with the irrigating solution. If the tube is not clean after flushing, discard it and connect a new sterile tube.

If the catheter and tubing are detached, as for irrigation, put a sterile cap over the tube end. To reattach the catheter, remove the cap from the tube and wipe the tube tip with an antiseptic swab.

Empty any drainage bag before it is three-fourths full. An overfull bag can cause urine to back up in the drainage tube.

Do not allow the tube end that enters the drainage bag to come into contact with anything other than the sterile inside of the drainage bag.

On a male patient, tape the catheter to the upper thigh so that the penis lies horizontally across the thigh. Alternate the catheter taping daily between one thigh and the other. Prevent a kink in the catheter by putting a piece of plastic tubing over the catheter at the site of taping.

Clean the patient's genitals with soap and water daily and more often if needed. Since matter tends to collect under the foreskin of an uncircumcized male, gently draw back the foreskin to clean that area.

Clear away any secretion around the point at which the catheter enters the body. Report crusts or irritations to the visiting nurse at once.

Wrap a gauze square dipped in Zephiran or another antiseptic solution around the tip of the penis and the catheter.

CONDOM URINARY DRAINAGE

A condom is a thin rubber sheath that fits snugly over the penis. The sheath is attached to one end of a length of rubber tubing. The other end of the tube is inserted into a drainage bag.

Whenever possible, doctors order condom drainage for male patients because the dangers of urinary infection are less than when indwelling catheters are used.

Applying a condom drainage system is not a sterile procedure, but cleanliness of equipment and method is essential. A patient may use the same rubber tubing and drainage bag over a period of several months. A regular routine for cleaning and sanitizing this equipment must be followed. The patient has two sets of equipment, which are alternated. One set is cleaned and sanitized while the second set is used.

A patient may wear one condom throughout a forty-eight-hour period. He should be checked often during every night and day, however, to see that the condom has not become twisted and that urine is draining. He should also be checked daily for signs of skin irritation or indications that the condom is no longer properly applied.

Enemas

An enema is the direction of a stream of fluid through the anus and into the rectum and large intestine. An enema is always ordered by the doctor. The kind of enema, the fluid or solution, and, sometimes, the quantity of fluid are part of the doctor's order. The doctor may order an enema for several reasons.

He may order a cleansing enema, such as an SSE (see below) or a Fleet, if the patient has not moved his bowels for a day or so.

He may order a tap water enema until the returns are clear to prepare a patient for X rays of the intestines.

Soapsuds Enema for a Bed Patient (SSE)

The temperature of the enema solution is very important. An older patient cannot tolerate as much heat as the normal adult patient. If the fluid is too hot it can burn the patient. If the enema is too cold, it will not effectively stimulate bowel movement. For an older patient, it should never be hotter than 105° F. (42° C.).

If the doctor does not specify the amount of solution, this can be determined by the condition and tolerance of the patient. A very ill patient is not given so much fluid that it causes strain or weakness. A person whose bowel is very distended with feces is unable to accept a large amount of fluid. In an older patient the anus or rectal opening is often lax and does not retain the fluid. Gently squeezing the buttocks around the enema tube and anus may allow more inflow. As an alternative, gently pressing a sanitary napkin against the anus during the inflow can increase the amount of retained fluid.

Equipment
    a strong wall hook or unplugged standing lamp base on which
        to hang the container of solution
    1 cup to 1½ quarts of water at 105° F. (42° C.)
    liquid soap (1 ounce to 1 pint of water)
    an enema can or a bag with rubber tubing and a tubing clamp
    a rectal tube
    a lubricant, such as Vaseline
    a small basin
    a bedpan and toilet paper
    a small washbasin with warm water
    a washcloth and towel

Adjust the hook or other holder to twelve or eighteen inches above the patient's hips.

Hang the can of solution.

Turn the patient onto his left side with his left arm behind his back and his right knee drawn high and relaxed on the bed.

Fasten the rectal tube onto the container tube and adapter.

Lubricate the rectal tube.

Unclamp the tubing to expel any air in the tube. Let it drain into the small basin.

Reclamp the tubing and insert the rectal tube into the anus using a gentle rotating motion.

Insert for three or four inches and hold in place.

Unclamp the tube and allow the solution to flow until the patient has taken all of it or until he protests.

Tell the patient to relax and take deep breaths through his mouth.

If the patient protests, pinch the tube for a second or two to stop the flow and allow him to rest. Then release the tube and lower the bag so that the fluid runs more slowly.

When finished, pinch the rectal tube near the anus and withdraw the tube slowly.

Clamp the tube and let any remaining fluid run into the emesis basin.

Disconnect the rectal tube from the adapter.

Put the rectal tube in the emesis basin.

Cover the patient and ask him to stay in position five or ten minutes or as long as possible.

When the patient is ready, help him onto the bedpan.

Elevate the head of the bed if permitted and desired.

Be sure the patient has the signal bell.

Leave the patient to expel the enema.

When the enema is expelled, remove the bedpan.

If the patient wipes himself, let him wash his hands in the basin of warm water.

If you wipe the patient, have him turn on his side again and you use the toilet paper and then the basin of warm water and a cloth to cleanse him.

Make the patient comfortable.

Remove the equipment from the bedside.

Empty the bedpan.

Observe and chart the returns.

Clean the equipment and sterilize anything that needs it.

Clear, or Tap Water, Enema

Follow the same procedure as for the soapsuds enema, omitting the soap. Repeat the procedure until the returns are clear.

Fleet Enemas

These are commercial, prepackaged, disposable enemas. There are two kinds. One is a cleansing enema; the other is an oil retention enema. The cleansing enema comes in two sizes, adult and child. These enemas are very popular because they are convenient and comfortable for both the patient and the person giving the enema. This is particularly true for the geriatric patient who cannot retain much fluid and the geriatric patient who is prone to constipation and fecal impaction. (The stool hardens and packs in the rectum and lower bowel so that the patient cannot expel the mass.)

Position the patient on his left side with his left arm behind his back and his right knee drawn high.

Remove the shield on the Fleet enema.

Insert the rectal tube into the anus.

Squeeze the bottle until the fluid is gone.

Remove the rectal tube from the anus.

Replace the shield on the rectal tube.

Throw the squeeze bottle with the tube into the waste container.

Have the patient retain the enema as long as possible. (Since very little fluid is given in a Fleet enema, the patient may retain the enema much longer than the soapsuds enema, sometimes for several hours.)

The mineral oil enema is given in the same way. If keeping a home record, note

the time the enema was given;
how it was accepted;
the name and amount of solution used;
the color, consistency, odor, and amount of the returns and the
presence of any unusual material such as blood or pus;
the effect upon the patient.

EXAMPLE: 4:30 P.M. — SSE (soapsuds enema) — about 1 quart — taken well and retained for 5 minutes.

Returns: a large amount of foul-smelling, thick, brown fluid with several very large, hard lumps of feces, streaked with mucus and red blood. The patient had pain when passing the feces but said he felt much better afterward.

Colostomy Care

In this operation a new opening of the large intestine is surgically created on the surface of the abdomen. Then the patient's bowels no longer move in the normal way, but through this opening. The opening is called a stoma. The patient has no control of his bowel movements through the stoma.

Colostomy Bag

This is a small, disposable, plastic bag with an adhesive cuff. The bag is placed over the stoma and the cuff adheres to the skin around the stoma. Then any fecal material is caught in the bag. The bag can be changed whenever necessary. Tincture of benzoin is sometimes put on the skin around the stoma to toughen the skin and to help the cuff adhere well. Special odor-control tablets are available for use in the bag.

Colostomy Irrigation Using a Douche Bag or Enema Can

It is necessary to irrigate (to flush or wash) a colostomy every two to three days or as the doctor orders. Special equipment is available for this procedure and, since the treatment is repeated many times, each patient usually has his own. It consists of an elastic waist belt with a hard, clear plastic bubble that fits over the stoma. The bubble has a small hole through which the irrigating catheter can be inserted into the colostomy opening. A length of disposable plastic tubing can be secured to the bottom of the bubble. The patient sits on the toilet with the tubing between his legs so that it drains into the toilet.

Equipment
   a colostomy irrigation set (belt, bubble, and sheath)
   a douche bag or can
   1 to 2 quarts of warm water
   a lubricant
   an adapter
   a small-sized catheter
   a clean colostomy bag
   tincture of benzoin
   a cotton-tipped applicator

Use the adapter to attach the catheter to the bag tubing.

Hold the bag or can twelve to eighteen inches above the stoma.

Clear the air from the tubing by letting some water run through it.

Pinch the catheter near the end.

Lubricate the catheter tip.

Insert the catheter through the bubble opening and then into the stoma six to eight inches.

Allow the water to run in. The water runs out almost at once and drains through the disposable tubing into the toilet. The water loosens and carries the feces with it.

After the water has run in, remove the catheter.

Allow the patient to remain on the toilet for fifteen to twenty minutes.

Remove and dispose of the plastic tubing.

Remove the belt and bubble.

Clean the stoma and the skin area around it.

Dry the skin area.

Apply tincture of benzoin to the skin area.

Use scissors to shape the opening of the bag to the size of the stoma.

Apply the bag to the stoma and skin area.

Help the patient off the toilet and make him comfortable.

Clean the irrigation set and ready it for the next irrigation.

If the patient is not allowed bathroom privileges, the irrigation may be done at his bed. The patient may either sit on the side of the bed or lie in a comfortable position. The belt is put on and the bubble placed over the stoma. One end of the disposable tubing is secured to the bubble and the other end placed in a bedpan at the bedside. Remember to follow the general rules for all treatments.

Since privacy is normal and helpful during bowel movements, the patient is usually taught to irrigate his colostomy, to change colostomy bags, and to care for the stoma. But if he is weak, confused, or otherwise unable, you will have to do it for him.

Put a clean gown on the patient.

Make the top of the bed.

Position the patient comfortably.

Use air deodorizer.

Remove the soiled laundry in the newspaper.

Remove all equipment. Clean, sanitize, and put away the patient's basin.

Colostomy Irrigation Using a Bulb Syringe

Instead of a bag and catheter, a bulb syringe tipped with a piece of flexible rubber or plastic tubing is used.

Equipment

a colostomy belt, bubble, and sheath

a bulb syringe with rubber or plastic tip

a pitcher with 24 ounces of water at 105° F. (42° C.)

a lubricant

Apply the colostomy bubble and belt.

Squeeze the bulb syringe to remove air before inserting the tip in water.

Draw water into the syringe.

Hold the tip of the syringe upward and press the bulb to remove remaining air.

Draw more water into the syringe.

Lubricate the tip and insert into the stoma for three to five inches.

Hold with the bulb up. Use both your thumbs to compress it, so that water flows in a steady stream.

Refill the bulb as necessary.

Avoid putting air into the stoma.

Have the patient take long, deep breaths during the irrigation.

Have the patient massage the area around the stoma during the irrigation.

After removing the sheath, clean the stoma and attach a clean colostomy bag.

When discharge ceases, remove the bag, clean the stoma, and apply a gauze dressing spread with lubricant. This can be held in place by an elastic girdle, shorts, or a clean colostomy bag.

Measuring Fluid Output

Fluids can leave the body through sweating, vomiting, liquid stools, heavy bleeding, etc. Most fluid leaves the body through urination. Sometimes a patient has a drainage tube inserted into a body opening.

Sweat, liquid stools, and blood loss are difficult to measure, although a descriptive note should be made on the patient's chart if any of these occur. EXAMPLE:

2:00 P.M. Perspiring lightly.
4:00 P.M. Sweating heavily. Patient's sheets and gown wet through.
10:00 A.M. Bowel movement. Large amount of dark brown liquid stool.

Vomiting (emesis) can be measured if it is liquid enough and if the patient has vomited into a container. Otherwise it must be estimated. EXAMPLE:

1:00 A.M. Emesis of about 180 cc. of partly digested food.
4:00 A.M. Emesis 6 ounces (360 cc.) of yellow liquid.
6:00 A.M. Incontinent of urine. Four bed pads soaked through.

Any drainage from the body through tubes into containers should be measured as needed or every eight hours and the amount recorded.

Home Method

Keep a plastic or glass measuring pitcher marked in ounces in the bathroom. Label the pitcher *Urine Only*. Use this pitcher to measure each voiding. Keep a record of these amounts. Change the amounts measured from ounces (oz.) into cubic centimeters (cc.). The pitcher should be thrown away when no longer needed by the patient. REMEMBER:

$$1 \text{ oz.} = 30 \text{ cc.}$$

Therefore, 6 oz. × 30 cc./oz. = 180 cc.

Catheterization

This procedure requires sterile technique. If the urine withdrawn by catheterization were needed for a specimen, it would be measured in a sterile pitcher and the amount noted on the output sheet before sending it to the lab. Only professional nurses or doctors should catheterize patients.

Urinary Drainage

Some disposable plastic bags used for Foley indwelling catheters or condom drainage have measures marked on them so you can read the amount in the bag before you empty it; if the bag is not marked, the urine in the bag must be emptied into a measuring pitcher. Each time the bag is emptied, the amount is written on the output sheet.

Specimens

Specimens are samples of body material or wastes that are sent to a laboratory for tests and examinations to find out whether the material is abnormal in certain respects.

Before Collecting a Specimen

Be sure you understand how to collect the specimen.

If in doubt, ask the doctor or nurse.

A proper container for a specimen is usually provided by the doctor or can be obtained from your druggist.

Be sure the patient's name, date, and type of specimen are on a label that you attach to the container.

After Collecting a Specimen

Chart the kind of specimen and the time of collection.

Urine Specimens

When collecting all urine specimens, note on the label if the patient has rectal or other bleeding that might enter the urine.

Routine. Have the patient void into a bedpan or directly into an unsterile but clean urine specimen bottle.

Midstream Urine. Have the patient start to void; then hold the specimen bottle to catch running urine.

Clean-Voided Urine. Clean the patient's genitals with sterile cotton balls and antiseptic solution. Then have the patient void into a sterile bedpan and transfer the urine to a sterile specimen bottle; or, after cleaning the genitals, catch a midstream sample in a sterile specimen bottle.

Twenty-Four-Hour Urine. Use a gallon bottle.

Label the bottle with the patient's name, address, and the hours of the collection. This bottle is usually kept in a refrigerator during the collection. EXAMPLE:

> Tom Jones, 417 E. 30th St. NYC.
> 7:00 A.M. to 7:00 A.M. 24-hr. collection urine
> (*The date marked is the one of the starting hour.*)

Have the patient void just before the start of the collection period and discard that voiding. Start the collection with the next voiding. Put the exact time of the discarded voiding on the collection label. EXAMPLE: 6:50 A.M.

Tell the patient that he is on a twenty-four-hour urine collection and that he must use his bedpan or urinal whenever he needs to void.

When he wants to have a bowel movement, he must void first or afterward into his specimen pan, but he should not void during the bowel movement, which would spoil the urine collection. He should have a separate pan for bowel movements. That pan should be marked BM.

Add the urine from each voiding to the gallon collection bottle.

At the end of the collection time, mix the urine in the bottle and measure the full amount.

If the total amount is required, put the urine back in the bottle. Your doctor will instruct you about this.

If portions, or aliquots, of the urine are required, measure out the amounts ordered into the right bottles and send them with the right laboratory report specimen sheets to the laboratory. Then discard the remaining urine.

Be sure the laboratory report and the chart are marked with

all the information on the collection bottle label;
the time of the last voiding that ended the specimen;
the total amount in cc.;
what amounts were sent to the laboratory;
what tests were to be done with each of these amounts.

Stool Specimen

Do not let the patient void into the bedpan being used to collect a stool specimen. Use the same technique as with a twenty-four-hour urine collection.

Use a disposable wooden blade to transfer feces from the bedpan to the specimen container.

Do not refrigerate the specimen unless a nurse tells you to do so. Most stool specimens should not be refrigerated.

11

Applying Heat and Cold

Heat treatment can be given internally by food, drink, enema, irrigation, etc., or externally by application to the outer body.

Wherever heat is given, it expands the blood vessels and increases the circulation to that area. So it is useful in bringing small infections to drain and in reducing congestion or inflammation. Heat soothes nerve endings and relieves certain pain. It helps relax muscle tension. External heat is given in three ways.

Dry heat is given by lamps, exposure to sunlight, electric pads and blankets, room heating, and hot water bottles.

Moist heat is given by soaks, compresses, steam inhalations, irrigations, baths, and chemical packs.

Medicinal heat is given by applying an irritant such as oil of wintergreen, liniment, or mustard plaster to the skin.

Before applying heat:

Learn the exact part of the body to be treated.

Be sure you understand in what way, for how long, and how often a treatment is to be given.

Be sure equipment is in good condition.

Follow the general rules for all treatments.

Position the patient in the most comfortable way that presents the part of the body to be treated.

Remove any dressings and discard them into a paper bag.

Use a bath thermometer to check the temperature of any hot solution before starting the treatment.

Electric Heat Lamps

Equipment
    a lamp
    an automatic timer
    skin lotion

Read the instructions about use of the lamp. Some hand types should be waved back and forth over the area to be treated.

Follow the general rules for all treatments.

Protect the patient's eyes if necessary.

Expose the area to be treated.

Plug in the lamp.

Position it at the correct height.

Set the timer for the exact time ordered by the doctor.

Turn on the lamp.

Start the timer.

Stay with the patient during the treatment and observe the area being treated.

Turn off the lamp when the timer goes off.

Stop the treatment and report at once if the skin shows any signs of burning or if the patient complains.

Apply skin lotion to the area after treatment.

Electric Pads and Blankets

Equipment
    an electric pad or blanket
    a clean cover (if a pad is used)
    a clean sheet (if a blanket is used)

Take care not to damage the heating element by folding or crushing the pad or blanket.

Put a clean cover on a pad before use; protect an electric blanket with a clean sheet.

Do not use a blanket or pad that is wet. (Wetness can cause shocks.)

Never use pins to fasten a pad or blanket in place. (Pins can damage the heating element.)

Heating pads should not be kept on continuously. Continuous use of heat interferes with the body's ability to respond to heat or cold.

Hot Water Bags

Equipment
   a hot water bag
   a cover, or a towel to cover the bag
   a bath thermometer

Test the water temperature. It should be 120° F. (47° C.). Do not test the temperature of running water. Draw the water into a container, then test it.

Half fill the bag with the tested water. (Too much water makes the bag heavy.)

Lay the bag flat on the sink or table; use the flat of your hand to press the bag gently until water appears on the neck. This removes air from the bag. Air in the bag makes it hard to manage and interferes with the heat radiation to the body.

Put the stopper on as tightly as possible.

Dry the bag well.

Test for leakage by holding the bag upside down.

Put the bag in a cover or wrap it in a towel. It should *never* be put directly on the skin as there is danger of burning.

Apply the bag to the proper area.

Remove the bag when the water cools.

Reapply as ordered.

AFTER USE
   Empty the water from the bag.
   Hang it upside down to drain.
   Leave the stopper off.
   To store, inflate the bag with air and put the stopper on. Lightly powder the outer surface of the bag.

Hot Compresses

Equipment
compress cloths (pieces of flannel or gauze)
hot pack machine or electric heating unit

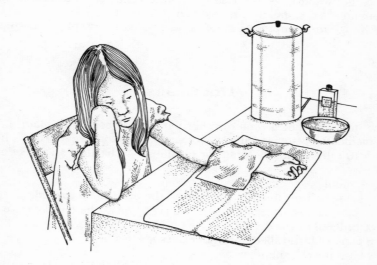

Setup for giving hot compresses

a bowl of the solution ordered by the doctor
towels
plastic wrap (such as Saran)
baby oil or petroleum jelly
a binder
hot water bottles, if permitted

Use this method if there is no break in the skin or drainage. If there is drainage, apply as in the method used for cold compresses.

Heat the compress cloths in the solution on the heating unit until they are as warm as you can handle.

While heating, prepare the patient.

Follow the general rules for all treatments.

Spread a towel under the area to be treated. Apply oil to the skin around the area.

Wring out the compress cloths as dry as possible. This keeps them hot longer and prevents their dripping on the patient.

Place the compress cloths over the area.

Cover the cloths with plastic wrap.

Put a binder on the area if needed to hold the compress in place.

Put a folded towel over the area to help retain the heat. Sometimes hot water bags are used to maintain the heat, but do not use them unless specifically directed to do so.

Change the compresses as often as needed to complete the treatment.

Hot Soaks

The immersion of a limb or other part of the body into plain, hot, or medicated water is called a hot soak. A doctor might order a hot soak to relieve muscle strain or tension or to localize an infection.

Equipment
    a basin or tub suited to the part of the body to be soaked
    pitcher or hot water at 110° F. (43° C.) or at the temperature
        ordered by the doctor
    a pad or plastic sheet for under the soak basin
    a bath towel or blanket
    another bath towel

Follow the general rules for all treatments.

Fill the soak basin less than half full.

Test the water temperature and correct if necessary.

Slowly introduce into the solution the body part to be soaked.

Cover the soaking part with the bath towel or blanket.

Check the time.

Allow the part to soak for the time ordered.

Watch the skin of the soaked area. Watch the general reaction of the patient.

Remove the soaked part from the basin.

Dry the part well.

If the water cools during the soak so that it is necessary to add more hot water, it should be drawn in the pitcher. Test the temperature and add it to the water in the soaking tub. Do not pour this water directly onto the skin.

Moist Hot Towels

Equipment
    two or more small-sized turkish towels
    a large double boiler
    a bath thermometer
    a plastic square
    a dry bath towel
    skin lotion

Wet towels and wring dry.
Fold into small pads.
Put folded towels in the top part of the double boiler.
Put water in the bottom part of the double boiler.
Put top in bottom part of double boiler.
Heat until towels are no warmer than 110° F. (43° C.).
Take the double boiler to the patient's bedside.
Prepare the patient.
Remove one moist towel and apply to the patient.
Cover the towel with the plastic square.
Cover the plastic with the dry towel.
Remove after ten minutes and apply the other moist towel in the same way.

Paraffin Bath or Dip

For hands and feet; used only for special conditions and when ordered by the doctor.

Equipment
    two ounces of mineral oil
    two ounces of paraffin
    a bath thermometer
    a double boiler large enough for the hand or foot to enter the
       top

Put the paraffin and mineral oil in the top of the double boiler.
Put the bath thermometer in the paraffin.
Put water in the bottom of the double boiler.
Put the boiler top inside the boiler bottom.
Heat over a low flame until the paraffin melts.
Watch the bath thermometer. Do not let the paraffin heat to more than 120° F. (47° C.) or it tends to burn.
Turn off the heat.
Remove the top of the boiler.
Let the paraffin cool to 110° F. (43° C.).
Dip the patient's hands (or feet) repeatedly, one at a time, into and out of the melted paraffin until a thick film has formed on both hands (or feet).
After thirty minutes, pull the paraffin off and replace it in the boiler top, to be used for the next treatment.

Hydrocollator Steam Pack

A hydrocollator steam pack is a closed fabric envelope that contains a substance that absorbs a great amount of water and retains heat for long periods of time. It is ideal for applying moist heat. No wringing is necessary and little dripping occurs. Packs are available in several sizes and are designed to fit body curves. They can be used over and over again.

Packs are heated by immersion in water at a temperature of from 110° to 120° F. (43° to 47° C.). A special electrically heated cabinet that automatically maintains water at the correct treatment temperature is used. This hydrocollator has frames to hold all packs that are not in use.

A pack must be covered with six layers of toweling before it is applied. Special six-layered hydrocollator covers are available and convenient. If a patient has thin, tender, or reddened skin, additional padding should be placed between the skin and the pack. Covers should be washed frequently.

Equipment
    a steam pack
    a six-layered cover
    a bath towel
    skin lotion

Check the temperature of the hydrocollator water.

Remove the correct size pack from the hydrocollator.

Place the pack inside the six-layered cover.

Place the pack on the folded bath towel.

Take the pack to the bedside.

Position the patient comfortably for the best application of the pack.

Place the pack with its cover on the correct part of the patient's body.

Hang the bath towel over a bedside chair or the foot of the bed.

Leave the pack in position on the patient for twenty to thirty minutes. Check the skin for irritation during first few minutes after application.

Remove the pack and place on the folded towel.

Place both on a bedside chair or stand.

Give skin care.

Reposition the patient.

Adjust bedclothes.

Take the pack and cover back to the hydrocollator machine.

Remove the cover and place on a drying rack.

Return the steam pack to the hydrocollator.

Cold contracts the blood vessels, decreases the circulation, and deadens nerve endings. It is used to control major infections such as appendicitis, to reduce swelling, and to deaden pain. There are three ways to apply external cold.

Dry cold is given by ice bags (caps or collars), air conditioning, and chemical packs.

Moist cold is given by soaks, compresses, baths, and irrigations.

Medicinal cold is sprayed on the skin. Cold is often applied in this fashion to anesthetize a small area for a short time.

Before applying cold:

Learn the exact part of the body to be treated.

Be sure you understand in what way, for how long, and how often a treatment is to be given.

Be sure equipment is in good condition.

Follow the general rules for all treatments.

Position the patient in the most comfortable way that presents the part of the body to be treated.

Remove any dressings and discard them into a paper bag.

Ice Bags (Caps or Collars)

Equipment
  an ice bag
  a cover for the bag
  ice chips (chip ice cubes easily by jabbing them with the open
     point of a large safety pin)

Fill the bag half full of ice chips. (More than half makes the bag
too heavy.)
  Squeeze the rest of the bag to expel air.
  Screw on the cap and test for leakage.
  Dry the bag well.
  Put on the ice bag cover. Do not apply a bag without a cover.
  Apply to the area to be treated.
  Remove when ice has melted.
  Reapply as directed.

After Use

  Remove the soiled cover and put it in the laundry.
  Take off the cap.
  Drain the bag and hang it upside down to dry.
  To store, inflate the bag with air. Screw on the cap. Keep in a
cool, dry place.

Cold Compresses

Equipment
  a tray
  a large basin half filled with crushed ice (Ice is never put di-
     rectly into a compress or soak solution, since a particle of
     ice can stick to the compress and get onto the skin.)
  a smaller basin with the ordered solution
  a protective pad
  a towel
  disposable plastic gloves, if needed

gauze compresses (a large pile)
a disposable paper bag

Follow the general rule for all treatments.
Place the protective pad under the area to be treated.
Cover the pad with the towel.
Position the area to be treated on the towel.
Place the small solution bowl into the large bowl with ice.
Put on the gloves.
Put the gauze compresses into the solution.
Wring out some of the compresses as dry as possible.
Stretch and place them on the area to be treated.
Remove them after a few minutes and discard them into the disposable paper bag.
Use new compresses and repeat the treatment until the time is up. (If there is no drainage, the same compresses can be reused.)

Cold Soaks

The immersion of a limb or other part of the body into cold, plain, or medicated water is called a cold soak.

Equipment
    a basin or tub suited to the part of the body to be soaked.
    a pitcher of water cooled with ice cubes
    a protective pad for under the soak basin
    a cotton blanket
    a bath towel

Follow the general rules for all treatments.
Fill the soak basin about half full with the chilled water.
Do not put ice directly into the soak water.
Slowly introduce into the water or solution the body part to be soaked.
Cover the rest of the patient's body with the cotton blanket. It is easy for a patient to chill if the soak involves a large body area. An additional blanket may be needed.
Check the time.
Allow the part to soak for the time ordered.
Observe the skin of the soaked part and the general body reaction

to the soak. Stop the soak if the skin becomes blue or the patient chilled.

When time is up, remove the soaked part from the basin.

Dry the part well.

Alcohol Sponge Bath

This type of bath is given to reduce general body temperature.

Equipment
  a washbasin
  a pint of lukewarm water at 90° F. (30° C.)
  a pint of rubbing alcohol
  a washcloth
  a bath towel
  a cotton blanket

Take the patient's temperature.

Pour the alcohol into the warm water.

Follow the general rules for all treatments.

Use a washcloth to sponge the patient's body in the same sequence as when giving a bath.

Expose the patient as little as possible. It is important to keep the patient covered to prevent chilling.

Pat rather than rub the skin to dry it.

Take the patient's temperature thirty minutes after the treatment.

12

Other Useful Techniques

Sterile Techniques, or Asepsis

Sterile technique and sterile materials are used whenever it is desirable to keep the danger of infection as low as possible.

For example, sterile technique is used for any operation, whether major or minor.

It is used in delivering a baby.

It is used in the examination and in the treatment of certain parts of the body, such as the urinary tract.

It is used in the examination and care of skin injuries and postoperative sites.

It is used when giving injections of any kind.

It is used when taking blood samples or whenever the skin is punctured or opened.

It is used in the collection of any specimens for culture.

To sterilize means to rid of germs. The three methods of sterilization in common use are

dry heat: an open flame or an oven;
moist heat: boiling or autoclaving (steam under pressure);
chemicals: antiseptic or germicidal solutions.

Time is a factor in sterilization, and the amount of time required depends on the method of sterilization, the size of the article to be sterilized, and on how contaminated the article is. (Contaminated means exposed to germs.)

SEE: Feeding (making formula).

General Rules

If opening a sterile package, touch only the outer, or unsterile, side of the wrapping with your hands.

If removing the lid of a sterile container, touch only the outside of the lid with your hands. Lay the lid down, inside up, and free from contact with unsterile objects.

The inside of a wrapping or a container is called a sterile field. Nothing unsterile should come near a sterile field. Even to reach across a sterile field contaminates it, or makes it unsterile.

Sterile forceps or gloves must be used to touch any part of, or any object within, a sterile field.

If the wrapping on a sterile bundle becomes wet, the bundle is considered contaminated.

If there is any doubt about the sterility of an article, it should be considered contaminated.

If pouring any antiseptic or sterile solution from a bottle, pour a small amount to discard. Then pour the amount to be used. The solution poured to discard cleans the lip of the container.

If pouring sterile solution from one container to another, do not touch the lips of the containers together.

Many sterile supplies are commercial disposables. Check the label of any package or container for the word *disposable* before discarding any part of it.

Check the wrapper of any disposable sterile package before using. If a wrapper is torn or punctured on a sterile disposable package, the package must not be used, but returned to the company for replacement.

HANDLING PICK-UP FORCEPS

Forceps are kept in a container filled with enough antiseptic solution to cover the prongs. The prongs should be in an open position in the solution.

Take hold of the forceps and close them while the prongs are still in the solution.

Draw the forceps straight up from the solution without touching the sides or top of the container.

Take care when removing forceps not to bump the sterile prongs against the unsterile upper part of the container.

Use the sterile prongs only to handle sterile things. Take care not to touch unsterile objects with them.

Return the forceps to the container during any time when you do not need to handle sterile things.

To replace forceps in their container, close and lower them straight down without touching the sides or top of the container.

Open the prongs after they are in the solution.

Wash your hands.

Check the label on the sterile glove package to be sure that you have the right-sized gloves.

Open the sterile glove package. Remove the powder packet and powder your hands.

Pick up the first glove by the cuff, touching only the inside of the glove.

Put it on the correct hand without touching any part of the outside.

Pick up the other glove with your gloved hand by slipping your fingers under the cuff.

Work that glove onto your hand, touching only the outside of the glove with your gloved hand.

When you have on both gloves you must take care to touch only sterile things.

Changing an Unsterile Dressing

For colostomy, hemorrhoids, vaginal drainage, etc.

Equipment
    a protective underpad
    a disposable bag (usually plastic)
    disposable gloves
    a clean dressing
    gauze squares
    a basin of warm water
    salve or ointment, if ordered
    a clean binder or tape to hold the dressings in place

Follow the general rules for all treatments.

Protect the bed with the underpad.

Put on the disposable gloves. This protects you from possible contact with germs.

Remove the old dressings and put them in the disposable bag. This prevents the possible spread of germs.

Use the gauze squares and warm water to clean the area.

Apply salve to the area, if ordered.

Put on the clean dressings.

Fasten them with tape or put on a binder.

Douche, or Vaginal Irrigation

Equipment

    1 to 1½ quarts of solution at 105° to 110° F. (40° C.)

    a douche bag

    a douche nozzle (sterile)

    a bedpan

    disposable gloves

    cotton balls

    lubricant

    a small basin

Prepare the ordered solution.

Follow the general rules for treatments.

Place the patient on her back with the knees flexed and separated and the soles of the feet flat against the mattress.

Drape the cotton blanket over the patient so that one corner is under her chin and the opposite corner is between her legs.

Arrange the other corners with one to cover each leg.

Draw the blanket up between the legs and onto the abdomen to expose the genitals.

Place the patient on the bedpan.

Hang the douche bag from a hook about a foot above the vagina.

Put on the gloves.

Connect the douche nozzle to the tubing.

Lubricate the nozzle (this is not always necessary).

Unclamp the tubing and allow the solution to run into the pan, then briefly over the external genitals. This cleanses them and prevents a transfer of germs from them into the vagina.

Insert the nozzle upward for three or four inches into the vagina while the solution is running. The upward direction is important since this allows easier entry.

Rotate the nozzle during the treatment; this better distributes the solution throughout the vagina. The solution drains from the vagina during the treatment.

When all the solution has been used, remove the nozzle from the vagina and place it in the small basin.

Use cotton balls to clean and dry the genitals.

Wipe once with each ball in one direction only, from front to anus (rectum).

Discard each ball into the emesis basin.

Remove the bedpan.

Remove the gloves and place them in the emesis basin.

After removing the equipment, sterilize and discard the douche nozzle and sterilize the bedpan.

Discard the gloves and cotton balls and clean the irrigating can, tubing, and basin with disinfectant solution. Rinse and return them to your storage place.

Binders

Binders are used
    to keep dressings in place;
    to give support;
    to limit movement;
    to apply pressure.

Except when put on to hold dressings in place, binders and restraints are used only when ordered by the doctor.

General Rules for Putting on a Binder

Never apply it so tight that it interferes with breathing or circulation.

Be sure it is firm enough to serve its purpose.

Be sure it is smooth and without wrinkles.

Be sure any dressing beneath the binder is in the right position.

Be careful when pinning a binder not to stick the patient.

T-Strap Binders

T-strap binders are often used to hold dressings in place on patients with rectal or urinal leaking. The binders are made of heavy muslin and are easy to launder. There are two types, a single strap and a double strap. The single-strap type is used on females, the double-strap type on males. Disposable binders are available from medical supply houses.

Equipment
    the right binder
    2 safety pins
    gauze dressings or genital pads
    a paper or plastic disposal bag

Remove the soiled binder.
Remove the soiled dressings and put them in the disposal bag.
Place the belt of the binder around the waist with the strap in the center of the back.
Position the dressing or genital pad.
Bring the strap or straps between the thighs and over the dressing.
Use the pins to secure the strap or straps to the belt.

Elastic Bandages

An elasticized pressure bandage is often used

to hold a dressing in place;
to support an injured limb;
to prevent an injured limb from swelling;
to prevent swelling of the feet and legs in patients with heart and kidney disease;
to prevent clots from forming in the leg veins after surgery;
to relieve pressure on varicose veins.

The bandages are available in hospitals and drugstores. They can be bought without prescription and come in widths of two, three, and four inches. The width used is determined by the size of the part to be wrapped. An elastic bandage should not be used on a geriatric patient unless ordered by a doctor.
SEE: Skin Care.

Applying an Elastic Bandage

Elevate the part to be bandaged; this lessens blood flow to the part.

Apply the bandage with a gentle, equalized tension and overlapping layers. Ask the patient if the bandage feels tight. It should feel comfortable but give support.

After a bandage is applied, watch for swelling and cold or blue skin below the wrapped area. These signs mean circulation interference, in which event the bandage should be removed and the condition reported to the doctor at once.

Remove the bandage at least once in every eight hours and leave it off for twenty minutes before reapplying. The skin should be carefully examined during these rest periods. Changes in the skin should be reported and skin care given before the bandage is replaced. Continuous use of the bandage can cause skin breakdown.

Wash the bandage often and dry it, without stretching, to renew the elasticity. Use a mild suds and rinse well. Geriatric patients often use elastic stockings rather than bandages. These should be cared for in the same way.

TO APPLY AN ELASTIC BANDAGE TO AN ANKLE

Place the end of the rolled bandage on top of the arch of the foot. Leave the toes exposed.

Wrap the arch twice in the same place to anchor the bandage.

Then wind the bandage around the ankle, back down to the foot, across the arch, and under the foot in a figure eight.

Repeat the figure eight, covering a new area of skin but overlapping the first figure eight. The heel is not wrapped unless so ordered.

Repeat the figure eight if necessary. Then continue wrapping the ankle and leg in spiral fashion, with each turn overlapping the last.

Adjust bandage so that the end of the last turn is on the outside of the leg.

Fasten the bandage with clips or safety pins. The bandage clips are placed on the outside of the leg so that they cannot catch on the other leg.

TO PUT ON AN ELASTIC OR SUPPORT STOCKING
Equipment
  a clean elastic stocking

Be sure the stocking is the right size for the patient.

Examine the stocking for holes. Do not use if a hole is present.

Test the stretch of the stocking for elasticity. Do not use it if the stretch is loose, or it does not return to its original shape after being stretched.

Roll the stocking to its toe end.
Elevate the patient's leg.
Put the toe of the stocking on the patient.
Unroll the stocking to cover the heel and foot.
Smooth the stocking foot so it is free of wrinkles.
Unroll the stocking to the knee.

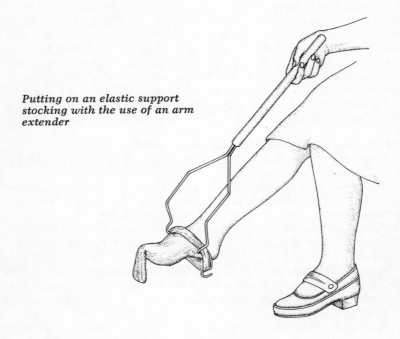

*Putting on an elastic support
stocking with the use of an arm
extender*

Smooth the stocking leg so it is free of wrinkles.
Unroll the stocking over the knee and thigh.
Smooth the stocking top so it is free of wrinkles.
Attach the top of the stocking to the girdle or garter belt. (Never use a leg garter on a patient; it interferes with the blood supply in the legs.)

Care for
Special
Conditions

13

The Aged, or Geriatric, Patient

Aging

Aging begins as soon as a baby is born. Even then, cells wear out and the body replaces them with new cells. In childhood and youth, the body's ability to make new cells is greater than the breakdown of old cells and so body growth occurs.

As life goes on, the ability to build cells and the breakdown of cells reaches a balance. Body growth stops but the body is maintained.

This balance lasts only a short while before breakdown of cells exceeds the body's ability to replace them. More and more signs of aging occur as the ability to make new cells decreases.

Aging, then, is a normal process that causes progressive impairments in the functioning of the body, mind, and emotional makeup of any person. These impairments force the older person to give up more and more of his independence. They may threaten his place of respect within his family, business, and social affairs.

As part of the aging process, a geriatric patient usually develops a number of chronic, or continuing, diseases, such as diabetes or arthritis. He must learn to accept these conditions and to live with them in the most satisfactory way. To do this, he may need treatments and may have to use special equipment. He may also have to learn new ways to take care of himself, may have to endure pain, and may be restricted from former pleasures. Any of these things can be discouraging. The geriatric patient, therefore, needs constant encouragement to meet the challenges of aging.

He seldom has the drive of youth to help him. The ambitions and competitive feelings of his younger years are often replaced by a withdrawal into himself. He may have a need for security and even for dependence. Recovery from a mild illness can be slowed by a reluctance to return to the struggles of life. Yet his desire to live is a strong force that you can use to encourage him.

You should be aware of the medical goals of geriatric care. They are

to maintain the structure of individual life;
to promote the ability to handle stress;
to help the patient reach and keep maximal physical and mental abilities.

You should also be aware of the emotional stress brought about by the conditions of aging. These are psychic blows and fears that affect the patient's health. They are

becoming dependent;
losing the respect of society;
losing self-respect;
losing the use of his senses, his abilities, and his mind;
being abandoned by loved ones;
adjusting to a new environment that requires him to give up some of his personal freedoms, belongings, position in his family and society, and habits, routines, and customs;
dying.

Observing the Patient

Although the technique for observing and recording symptoms are the same for any patient, regardless of age, a definition of normal health always depends on age. What is normal for a two-year-old is not normal for an adult. What is normal for an adult is not normal for an old person.

The normal, expected body behavior of an old person is one of gradual breakdown and decreasing function. A definition of health in a geriatric person, therefore, must be based on ability to function rather than on perfection of function.

Also, signs, degrees, and rates of aging differ from one person to another and from one part of the same body to another. One man may develop many wrinkles and be bald at forty, while another may have few wrinkles and a full head of gray hair at seventy. A person of fifty may have the stomach of a forty-year-old, the heart of a sixty-year-old, and the liver of an eighty-year-old. Nearly every old person has one or more chronic health problems.

Then, too, it is important to remember that signs of aging are seldom sudden or dramatic. In fact, they develop so slowly that, unless deliberately sought, they can be overlooked. Early notice of a sign of aging allows for better treatment and can prevent or slow disability.

It is also important to remember that aging lowers resistance to any illness. A geriatric patient is more prone to acute diseases such as colds, flus, and intestinal infections. Acute disease affects him more severely and he is slower to recover.

In order to observe a geriatric patient, you must

be alert to recognize general signs of aging;
be familiar with the patient's specific history of aging and be alert for changes;
be alert for signs of acute illness.

Signs of Aging

Bones grow brittle and break easily. Joints become painful and stiff, restricting motion.

Blood circulation slows and the heart enlarges. Hardening occurs in some blood vessel walls. Clots tend to form in blood vessels. Varicose veins and ulcers are common. The strain on the blood vessels causes some to break. High or low blood pressure may develop.

Nerves react slower, and the person therefore responds more slowly to any stimulation of the senses. Interests change from active affairs to quieter ones. Trembling may occur. The mind may become easily confused. The person is apt to forget recent happenings and to remember the past with clarity. Speech may become repetitious or difficult.

Teeth may decay and the gums recede and become infected. The desire for food may lessen. Bowel function slows and movements become difficult. Disorders such as diabetes, gallstones, and ulcers may appear. Hemorrhoids may develop. The anus may lose muscle tone and control of bowel function lessen.

The elasticity of the lungs lessens. Breathing may become difficult. Coughing may be frequent. Colds, flus, and upper respiratory infections last longer and require more care.

The kidneys may not function well. The bladder sphincter muscle may lose control and the person may need to urinate often or may dribble urine. Bladder infections may occur.

Sexual interest decreases. The male may develop prostate trouble that can interfere with his ability to void. Glandular slowdown causes figure changes and can trigger depression.

The skin loses elasticity and dries, bruises, wrinkles, infects easily, and heals slowly. Pressure sores or decubitus ulcers easily develop.

Hair thins, dries, and turns gray.

Hearing ability lessens.

The sight blurs, or becomes restricted. Cataracts may form and glaucoma may develop.

Rest and sleep requirements change. The person may need to rest more often after less exertion. He may sleep for shorter periods but need frequent naps.

Patient Care

The care of a geriatric patient has three separate but interrelated parts:

> self-care
> activities
> nursing care

Self-Care

Some people think that showing concern for an elderly person means relieving him of all responsibilities and efforts. They argue that an old person has earned the right to do nothing and to have others wait on him. These people mean well, but they are wrong to confuse care with unnecessary service.

A geriatric patient should not exhaust himself, and he should have as much help as he needs. The word to remember is *needs*. He needs only that amount of help without which he could not function. Unnecessary assistance can harm him.

In self-care, the patient is provided with needed physical activity and with important feelings of independence and pride. Self-care helps him to remain alert to his surroundings and to prolong his life.

To encourage and maintain the patient's ability to perform self-care, his doctor orders a regular program of physical therapy. If the patient is physically handicapped, the doctor orders special equipment, such as a brace, walker, or wheelchair, that will keep the patient active. The doctor also orders training in activities of daily living, through which the patient learns new ways to help himself function. The doctor may order adaptive equipment that enables the patient to feed, dress, groom, and help himself in the bathroom.

Activities

A patient also needs other activities. He should have work to do that carries over from one day to the next. He should have opportunities to learn, and he should have a social and recreational life.

Occupational therapy trains the patient for and provides work. Depending on a patient's ability and interests, his participation in occupational therapy may range from full-time employment at a regular job to a few minutes spent on a simple craft.

Many patients are able to operate full-time businesses from their homes. Many learn new hobbies. Educational television, home study courses, and technical and professional magazines offer interesting learning experiences. Some cities have special programs of home study with teachers who visit in the homes.

Certainly, when able, the patient should have chores that contribute to family life. These can be as simple as stringing beans, peeling potatoes, or darning socks. Or they might be more complicated, such as helping a child with homework or planning household menus for the week.

Occupational therapy can be shared recreation for the family. Learning new games, working with craft materials, or making useful things such as party favors for a birthday can be fun for all.

The intent of all activities is to involve the patient as much as possible, to keep him interested, to keep him active, and to keep him in the mainstream of life.

Remotivation is the process of renewing a person's urge to live and stimulating his desire to be active and to learn.

Resocialization is the process of renewing a person's awareness of others and stimulating his desire and ability to participate in groups.

Both remotivation and resocialization are necessary on a daily, hour-to-hour basis throughout the lifetime of every person, from the loving encouragement of a baby's first steps, to the rewarded successes of adult life. The geriatric patient, though still in need of frequent encouragement, usually receives less and less.

Aging reduces the contact between a geriatric patient and the world. Communication problems, such as faulty vision, failing hearing and brain damage, make social relationships difficult. Lessening ability to move about, disease, and lowered income restrict an older person's activities. Deaths of family members and long-time friends deprive him of those who knew him best and shared his life and interests.

Because of these things and because the aging mind tends to forget present events and to recall the past, a patient often withdraws into himself, becomes lonely, depressed, and loses interest in life. If allowed to continue in this state of mind, he deteriorates into total dependency and untimely death.

It is important then that a geriatric patient be stimulated into activities and social relationships. It is one of the main duties of all persons involved in the care of an older person.

Nursing Care

Nursing is the last part of a geriatric care plan to be mentioned here. This does not mean that nursing is less important than self-care or activities. It does mean that the first duty in geriatric nursing is to cooperate with and enforce self-care and activity programs.

Dealing with Changing Needs

Skeletal

Prevent tripping and falling by following the usual safety measures. SEE: Safety in Chapter I.

Have the patient wear well-made, well-fitting shoes.

Keep stairways, halls, and rooms free of obstacles.

Provide good lighting.

Provide handrails wherever necessary, e.g., in the tub or shower.

Use bedrails when necessary.

Use safety seat straps and binders on chairs and wheelchairs.

Use walking aids ordered by the doctor, such as braces, canes, and walkers.

Blood Circulation

Keep the patient as active as possible.

Keep the person dry and warm.

Stimulate circulation with mild active and passive exercises.

Do not permit the patient to wear constricting clothes such as garters, tight brassieres, girdles, or tight collars.

Give good skin care.

Elevate the person's feet when he rests.

Nervous System

Set a slower pace for yourself. Bustling activity irritates the older person. Never rush him or show impatience at his slowness.

See that the patient gets as much rest, air, exercise, and diversion as he can.

See that the patient eats well and in pleasant surroundings.

Build a "care" plan around the patient's interests such as special television programs, bridge games, and car rides.

Listen to everything the patient has to tell you. If he repeats, ignore the repetitions and never treat him as you would a child.

Be careful when applying heat of any kind. Lowered sensitivity may not warn the patient that he is being burned.

Digestive System

See that regular dental care is given.

Provide dentures when needed.

Keep the patient's mouth clean and fresh.

Feed him simple foods.

Avoid spices and strong seasonings.

Follow orders for any special diet.

Keep his bowels in good working condition by whatever means the doctor may order.

Respiratory System

Allow the patient to rest in a position that is easy for breathing.

See that air is clean and fresh.

Keep nose and throat passages clean.

Provide tissues for discharges and a handy disposal bag.

Provide a sputum cup if necessary.

Urinary System

See that the patient drinks sufficient fluids.
Observe the patient's urine for changes in color and quantity.
Keep the patient's pubic area clean and free of odor.
Provide padding for dribbling urine. Change it frequently.
Provide for incontinence. SEE: pages 164–167.
Watch urinary drainage bags.

Skin

Keep patient as active as possible.
Give frequent baths and skin care.
Use lotion on the body skin.
Use very little soap.
Take care of cuts and scratches at once.
Take care when cutting the patient's nails not to injure the skin.
Use padding on furniture to avoid bruises and bumps.
Report to the doctor any sign of skin breakdown.
Use an electric razor to prevent cuts.

Hair

Wash and brush the patient's hair often.
Use oil on the hair.
Arrange the hair attractively.

Hearing

Speak in a loud, clear voice.
Teach family and visitors to face the person and speak clearly and slowly.
If the person uses a hearing aid, see that extra batteries are on hand. When the patient is not wearing the aid, place it within his easy reach.

Sight

Provide good lighting.
Provide regular eye examinations.
Provide rest periods for the eyes.
See that the patient's glasses are always within his reach.

Take precautions against possible accidents. Fence stairways, use nightlights, and the like.

Rest and Sleep

See that the patient has quiet and solitary periods to meet his rest and sleep needs.

The Patient's Diet

A doctor considers many things before ordering a diet for a geriatric patient. Some of the main considerations are

whether the patient has one or more chronic diseases;
the patient's blood chemistry and general health;
the patient's nutritional needs;
the patient's decreased digestive and intestinal function;
the patient's weight;
the patient's eating habits, tastes, and religious restrictions.

Chronic disease is always the first consideration. Diabetes, hypertension (high blood pressure), and many other conditions can be controlled only by special diets.

A patient's blood chemistry reveals much about the health of his body. Abnormal readings on blood tests are causes for a doctor to make adjustments in a patient's diet. For example, if the blood potassium reading were low, a doctor might order a low-salt diet and increased intake of specific foods, such as orange juice, that are rich in potassium.

A geriatric patient requires foods from the same basic nutritional groups as any adult. He needs meat or other protein, fruits and vegetables, bread and cereal, and dairy products. As aging decreases his activity, however, he may require decreasing total food intake. He also may need more protein to help repair tissues affected by the increasing cellular destruction of aging, more fruits and vegetables to stimulate bowel function, additional vitamins and minerals in tablet or capsule form, alcohol or coffee for general stimulation, or no coffee or alcohol for decreased stimulation.

Many problems can result from decreased digestive and intestinal function, and the doctor must consider the patient's specific ones. For example, a patient may have ill-fitting false teeth due to gum shrinkage, be unable to digest milk, have a history of diverticulitis (a pocket in the intestinal tract that is subject to frequent infection), and suffer from constipation. For such a patient, the doctor might order a soft diet, limited intake of milk products, no spices or roughage, and daily prune juices.

Most geriatricians agree that an older person should tend to be thin. Excess weight strains the heart and other organs and interferes with physical activity. No caloric restrictions are put on the patient's diet unless he is overweight or gaining weight. Then the doctor might order a diet with limited intake of fats and carbohydrates (sugars and starches).

As a person grows older, his eating habits sometimes change. He seems to eat less at a meal but to require food more often than three times a day. Doctors often recommend frequent, smaller meals — five or six meals instead of three. The person should be able to select foods that he likes whenever they fill his special dietary requirements.

Taking the Patient's Temperature

Under normal circumstances a geriatric patient seldom requires his temperature to be taken more often than once a week. A patient under constant medical supervision may need a daily or more frequent reading. A patient with an acute illness such as the flu may require a reading every four hours. Any patient with an elevated temperature should have frequent temperature checks. Any person who complains of feeling unusually ill should have an immediate temperature check.

Aging interferes with the body's ability to regulate its temperature. The thermometer readings of older people often register lower than the normal that is marked on the thermometer. This is not usually a cause for concern. However, any reading lower than 97° F. (36° C.) by mouth, 98° F. (37° C.) by rectum, and 96° F. (35° C.) by axilla should be reported to the doctor at once.

14

Arthritis

Arthritis is a chronic disease that causes inflammation and pain in the joints and can affect anyone at any age. It can affect fingers, wrists, elbows, shoulders, the spinal vertebrae, hips, knees, ankles, and toes. The cause is unknown, although two types of arthritis are recognized: rheumatoid arthritis and osteoarthritis.

Most older people suffer periodic attacks of arthritis, but with some the disease is progressive. The patient experiences intense pain and joint changes that make movement difficult.

Such a patient may require a great deal of personal attention and nursing care. Because his movements are slow and painful, nursing care may take longer than with another patient. Then, too, the personality of the arthritic patient is often affected by the disease. He may be very emotional, depressed, complaining, and demanding.

His attitude, combined with his slowness, can be very irritating unless you remind yourself that he does not want to be the way he is. He cannot change. You must always be calm, patient, kind, and gentle. Try to imagine how his pain and frustration must feel. Remember how much he needs you.

Setting Up a Unit for the Patient

Place the bed where it isn't near a window or other source of draft.

The unit should include
an adjustable bed;

a hinged bedboard to allow for elevating the head of the bed;
a firm mattress covered with a foam mattress;
a flat head pillow;
a covered footboard;
a comfortable armchair with raised seat level.

Medication

Arthritic patients often receive aspirin or a pain medicine containing it. Aspirin should be given with milk or other food. This medicine often causes sweating. The patient's clothing should be changed when sweating occurs, and care should be given to avoid drafts.

Rest

An important part of the care plan is sufficient rest. The patient should have a quiet, regular routine that includes as much occupational and recreational therapy as he enjoys. The patient should not become overtired, excited, or emotional, however.

Night bed rest should be eight to ten hours.

Daytime bed rest — two daily hour-long periods — should be required.

Positioning

Use a firm mattress in bed.

See that the spine and the head are in a straight line.

Adaptive Equipment

The arthritic patient often requires walking aids: special shoes, a cane or Loftstrand crutch, or a walker. When the disease is severe and deforming, he may need a wheelchair. However, every effort should be made to keep him as mobile as possible and to prevent permanent stiffness of joints. The disease has acute periods during which one or more joints become more intensely inflamed. When these periods occur, the doctor may order a temporary rest for the joint. For example, an arm sling may be ordered to rest the arm and shoulder until the acute stage passes.

Food and Fluid

A good diet for arthritics furnishes all the essentials for proper nourishment but keeps the patient's weight at a minimum. Excess weight aggravates arthritis. Since weight is an individual condition, and arthritics often require other dietary specifications, the doctor orders a diet to suit the patient. EXAMPLE: An overweight arthritic patient may have high blood pressure and diabetes. In that case, the doctor would order a low-calorie, salt-free, and sugar-free diet.

The arthritic patient often needs encouragement to eat. If eating involves pain, the patient tends to eat less and to select food from his meal. He may also reject or pick at food when emotional. By doing so, he may change the nutritional balance of his diet. Close watch should be taken of the patient's eating pattern, and changes in the patient's food intake reported to the doctor.

Many ADL aids are available to help the patient with arthritis involving the arm and hand. The physical therapist and ADL nurse usually work with the patient to discover which ADL aids are best for him. See that the patient uses the prescribed feeding aid. Although it may appear easier to feed him, you would be doing him harm by doing so if a feeding device has been ordered.

Bowel Control

Sitting on the toilet, commode, or bedpan often involves pain for this patient, and he may tend to put off bowel movements until fecal impaction occurs. Every effort should be made to make the patient as comfortable as possible while he has a bowel movement. A raised toilet seat and correct bedpan positioning are two of the many ways to help.

A close watch should be kept on the patient's bowel movements and changes reported. The doctor usually orders laxatives and enemas as needed to keep the bowels in good working condition.

Rehabilitation Through ADL Training

There is a limit to how much a patient with progressive arthritis can be rehabilitated. He may also require periodic rehabilitation to meet his decreasing abilities with different devices. He should be kept as self-sufficient as possible, however, and encouraged in self-care. Changes in his ability to use ADL devices and to perform daily activities should be reported to the doctor.

Physical Therapy

Specific passive and active range of motion (ROM) exercises may be ordered. Unless the doctor specifies the number, each exercise should be done no more than five times during one exercise period. Heat is helpful in relieving pain and stiffness. Only moist heat, however, should be used. Methods of heat therapy often used include thirty-minute tub baths in water at 105° F. (40.5° C.), hydrocollator pads, paraffin baths, contrast baths, and moist hot towels.

15

Communicable Disease and Isolation Technique

Communicable disease is illness caused by the spread of germs from an infected person to a well person.

Such germs can be transmitted through cough droplets; contact with a bowel movement; contamination of water, food, or milk; contact with skin lesions or blood; inhalation of dust containing germs; and the use of contaminated needles and syringes. Contaminated means "in the presence of germs."

A person or animal on whom a germ lives is called a *host*. A person with a cold would be a host because he carries the cold germs and has symptoms of a cold.

A person or animal who carries a germ but does not have symptoms of the disease is called a *carrier*.

Some diseases can be transmitted but are not contagious. These are called *infectious* diseases. Venereal diseases are infectious.

Diseases that spread easily from sick to well persons are called *contagious* diseases. Mumps and measles are contagious.

Isolation technique involves the separation of a person and his belongings from contact with others in order to prevent the spread of a communicable disease.

Even though a patient on isolation care is set apart from others and special precautions and techniques are used in caring for him, he should receive as excellent care as any other patient.

Preventing the Spread of Disease

The decision concerning the degree of isolation technique that is necessary depends on how infectious or contagious a disease might be, the condition of the patient, and the policy of the individual hospital or doctor.

Isolation technique has long been used in such illnesses as tuberculosis, hepatitis, tetanus, and wound infections, as well as childhood diseases such as measles and mumps.

Today, it is also used in the care of patients before and after organ transplants. A transplant patient requires drugs that prevent his body from rejecting the transplant. However, these drugs also reduce his body's ability to resist infections. Isolation technique is used to prevent germs from being carried to these patients. This same protective isolation is used in hospital nurseries.

The most important control of any disease, inside or outside of isolation technique, is maintained by frequent and careful hand washing. You should wash your hands before and after caring for any patient or his belongings. But isolation technique goes further than hand washing.

The patient is placed in a room or area by himself.

The room or area should be near a sink, supplied with a disinfectant soap, such as pHisoHex, and paper towels.

Anyone entering the room should wash his hands before entering and after leaving.

Anyone entering the room should wear a hospital gown over his regular clothing and a mask that covers his nose and mouth.

Waste disposal is handled in a special way, apart from regular garbage.

All equipment used in the care of the patient is kept apart from use by others or sterilized before use by others.

Plastic gloves are worn when it is necessary to touch very contaminated material.

Soiled laundry is handled apart from other linen.

Isolation Procedures

Setting Up

Put the patient in his own room with a private bath, if possible.
Place a table just outside the entrance to the unit or room.

Put supplies of clean isolation gowns, masks, and gloves on the
table. Add a supply of clean disposable towels.

Attach a laundry bag for soiled gowns to the side of the table.
Place a wastebasket with a plastic bag liner next to the table.

Place a clothes rack next to the table.

Put a large sign on the doorway, or unit entrance, that reads
ISOLATION.

Set up a food tray and dishes for use by the patient only. Mark
the tray in the same way as the bedside equipment. Cover the tray
with a clean disposable towel.

Disposable gowns are available at medical supply houses. Disposable plastic gloves and masks are found in drugstores.

A basin for hand washing can be put on the supply table if a sink
is not nearby.

If a basin is used, a large pitcher containing water should also be
kept on the supply table. Keep the pitcher covered with a clean, dry,
disposable towel. A disinfecting agent, such as bleach or alcohol,
can be added to the water in the pitcher.

A clean mask is used by each person entering an isolation room.
Disposable masks are most commonly used; these can be purchased
at any drugstore.

Washing Your Hands and Arms

Equipment
   paper towels
   soap
   running water
   orange stick

Use a paper towel to turn on the water. This prevents your touching the faucet with contaminated hands.

Wet your hands and soap them well.

Rub the palms together ten times.

Use the palm of one hand to wash the back of the other hand. Rub ten times.

Reverse this position and rub ten times.

Interlace the fingers of both hands. Rub back and forth ten times.

Cup one thumb in the other hand. Rub up and down ten times.

Reverse this position and rub ten times.

Clean under the nails of one hand with a nail from the other hand or orange stick.

Reverse this position and clean.

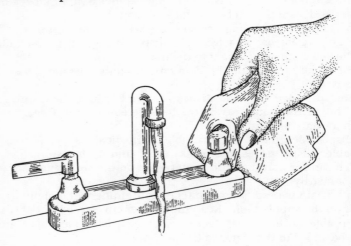

Using a paper towel to handle faucets prevents germ spread.

Rinse your hands by holding the fingers in a downward direction under the running water.

Soap your hands again.

Encircle one wrist with the other hand.

Move that hand upward in a spiral fashion to wash the wrist and arm to the elbow.

Reverse your hand positions to wash the other arm.

Rinse your arms by holding the hand upward so that the water runs off the elbow.

Use paper towels to dry hands and arms.

Use a paper towel to turn off the water.

Feeding the Patient

Take a regular tray of food from the kitchen to the table outside the entrance door to the patient's room.

Set it next to the patient's isolation food tray.

Remove the cover from the patient's isolation tray and dispose of the cover.

Transfer the food from the regular dishes to the patient's isolation dishes without touching anything on the isolation tray.

Put on a gown and mask.

Serve the patient's food trays as you would to any other patient.

When the patient is done with his meal, wash the dishes at the patient's sink, dry them, and put them back on his isolation tray.

Return the tray to the table outside the entrance to the room.

Remove your isolation gown and mask.

Cover the tray with a clean cover.

Return the uncontaminated tray to the kitchen.

Caring for Waste by Double Bagging

Wear an isolation gown and a mask.

Line the trash cans in the room with heavy plastic bags.

To empty, remove the bag and tie the top.

Have an uncontaminated bag or box ready outside the room entrance.

Put the tied plastic trash bag into the uncontaminated bag or box.

Touch only the inside of the uncontaminated bag or box.

Remove isolation gown and mask.

Touch only the outside of the second bag or box.

Tie or close this bag or box.

Wash your hands again.

Tag the bag or box with an ISOLATION sign.

Caring for Linen

At home, soiled isolation linen should be kept in a separate bag and washed apart from other household linens. A germicide, or germ-killing agent, should be used during the laundry process. Clean linen should be kept only for isolation-room use until the isolation period is ended. Then all linens used in the isolation room should, before laundering, be soaked for a half hour in a germicide. If possible, they should be dried by sunlight and air.

Caring for Equipment

At home, equipment must also be set aside from use by the household. When the household toilet is used to empty the bedpan

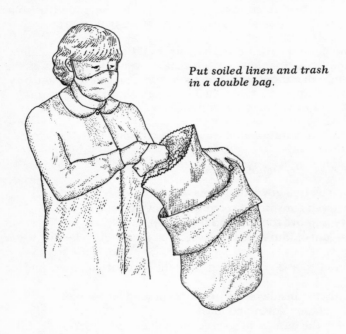

Put soiled linen and trash in a double bag.

it must be disinfected after each use. If the patient uses the family bathroom, it must be disinfected after each use.

When isolation ends, all equipment must be cleaned and sterilized thoroughly before use by others.

Caring for a Room When Isolation Ends

Wear isolation gown and mask.

Strip the room of all washable articles. Soak these in germicide and then wash. Dry them in sun and air, if possible.

Throw away any articles such as books, toothpaste, toothbrush, tissues, magazines, or toilet paper that have been in the isolation area and so are contaminated. Use the isolation waste technique of double bagging.

Disinfect the bed and entire unit.

Disinfectant bombs are available at drugstores. One of these can be set off in the room after all the doors and windows are closed. The bomb smokes for a period of several hours and decontaminates the room and its furnishings. This process is called *fumigation.*

Close the doors and open the windows to air the room for twenty-four hours.

Communicable Diseases

Chicken Pox

Cause: Virus contracted through direct contact with a breath droplet from an infected person.

Incubation period: There is a period of ten to twenty-one days between the time of first contact and the appearance of the first symptoms.

Signs: Small pimples, which become blisters and then scabs, appear on all parts of the body. The rash is very itchy. The temperature is elevated.

Care: Relieve the itching with cornstarch or bicarbonate of soda baths. Do not rub the skin. Keep the patient from scratching. Follow the doctor's orders for medication, rest, and diet.

The Common Cold

Cause: Virus.
Signs: Sneezing, coughing, fullness in the head.
Care: Follow the doctor's orders. It usually lasts ten days.

Conjunctivitis, or Pink Eye

Cause: Bacteria and virus from direct or indirect contact. Spreads rapidly from one eye to another and from one person to another.

Signs: Reddened whites of the eyes; pus drainage from eye; crusty eyelids, tears, itching, or burning.

Care: Frequent gentle wiping of affected eye to remove drainage.

Use a tissue once only and dispose immediately to prevent anyone's further contact with it.

Only the patient should use his towel and washcloth.

Should be seen by the doctor.

Hepatitis

Cause: Virus spread through contaminated food or water or by blood contact with an infected object (such as a needle).

Signs: Sudden nausea, vomiting, fever, skin itching, yellow skin color, air hunger.

Care: Doctor's care. Bed rest for three to six weeks. High protein, high starch diet. Precautions with bowel movements to prevent contamination of food or water and consequent spread of the disease.

Impetigo

Cause: Staphylococcus germ.

Signs: Small, pus-filled blisters appear on the face, ears, hands, and other body parts. They spread rapidly, form in clusters, and are highly contagious.

Care: Preventive cleanliness against spread of eruption. Keep the nails clipped short to prevent scratching. Follow the doctor's orders.

Influenza

Cause: Specific virus.

Signs: Cold symptoms, fever, sore throat, intestinal cramps, diarrhea, general weakness.

Care: Rest, force drinking fluids, keep warm, aspirin; follow doctor's orders.

Measles, German

Cause: Virus contracted through direct contact with a breath droplet from an infected person.

Incubation period: There is a period of fourteen to twenty-one days between the time of first contact and the appearance of the first symptom.

Signs: Same as for red measles but much milder.

Care: Same as for red measles but rash disappears after third or fourth day.

DANGER! Women who contact the disease during the first three months of pregnancy may bear children deformed by the disease. Check with your doctor.

Measles, Red or Black

Cause: Virus contracted through direct contact with a breath droplet from an infected person.

Incubation period: There is a period of seven to fourteen days between the time of first contact and the appearance of the first symptoms.

Signs: Cold symptoms for two or three days; flat, pink spots start behind the ears and spread to cover the body; very high fever; itchy, reddened, watery eyes.

Care: Follow the doctor's orders. Isolate the patient from other children and elderly family members. Keep the child in bed in a warm, but not overheated, draft-free room. The room should be kept somewhat darkened and the child discouraged from reading or watching TV if light irritates the eyes. Force fluids. Give mouth care three times daily. Keep the body clean. Be alert for, and try to prevent, complications such as ear abscess, bronchitis, pneumonia. The rash lasts ten to fourteen days.

Mumps

Cause: Virus contracted through direct contact with a breath droplet from an infected person.

Incubation period: There is a period of twelve to twenty-four days between the time of first contact and the appearance of the first symptoms.

Signs: Swelling of the saliva-producing glands located under the ears and jaw, pain in the ear on swallowing, temperature elevated for two or three days, poor appetite, inability to swallow acid foods such as orange juice, pickles, vinegar.

Care: Isolate the patient. Follow the doctor's orders. Keep the patient comfortable. Force fluids but give nonacid juices.

DANGER! Males who contract the diseases as adults may have changes in sperm strength.

Scarlet Fever

Cause: Streptococcus infection through contact with infected person or materials.

Signs: Fever, sore throat, strawberry-colored tongue, rash over entire body.

Care: Follow the doctor's orders. Isolate the patient. Force fluids. Keep skin clean. Keep the patient in bed.

DANGER! Scarlet fever often leads to such complications as rheumatic fever, kidney disease, ear infection, and blood poisoning.

Strep Throat

Cause: Streptococcus infection.

Signs: Very sore throat with or without fever. White spots on throat.

Care: Follow the doctor's orders. Isolate the patient. Force fluids. Keep skin clean. Keep the patient in bed.

Thrush

Cause: Fungus infection of the membrane of the mouth. It is spread through contact with the infection, and is highly contagious.

Signs: White patches that look like milk curds appear on the gums, tongue, the back of the throat, and the lining of the mouth.

Care: Prevent by strict cleanliness. But if it appears, follow the doctor's orders. Give sterile water by mouth after every feeding. Never rub the sores or try to wash out the mouth.

Whooping Cough

Cause: Bacillus germ contracted through direct contact with a breath droplet from an infected person.

Incubation period: There is a period of seven to ten days between the time of first contact with the disease and the appearance of the first symptoms.

DANGER! Can be fatal for newborns.

Signs: Cough with whooping sound on inspiration, gagging, vomiting. The discomfort is worse at night.

Care: Isolation technique. Follow the doctor's orders. Support the patient during coughing attacks; give frequent small feedings of easily swallowed foods. Provide fresh air but no drafts.

16

Death and Dying

Not so long ago, few patients were allowed to discuss dying and death. Doctors, nursing personnel and families conspired to hide from patients the deadly possibilities of illness. However, in recent years researchers have studied the psychological effects of dying and death upon patients and their families. These researchers have found that except in sudden death, a dying person usually goes through five progressive emotional stages other than fear and anxiety.

When confronted with death, a person's first reaction is denial. It is very difficult for one to imagine his own death. Death seems to be something that happens to others. A person thinks, "It can't happen to me!"

After he realizes that he *can* die, his second reaction is anger. He feels singled out for misery. He asks, "Why me?" And then he defies death. He says, "I won't die!"

When death continues to threaten, the person enters a third stage. He begins to bargain for his life. He says such things as, "I'm going to give up all my bad habits if I get well!" Or, "If I get out of this, I'm going to give all my money to benefit others."

But as the dying process goes on, the patient has a fourth reaction. He becomes very depressed. At first the depression is a form of grief because he must leave life. The patient may cry, withdraw from the attentions of family and friends, or even become hostile to them. He may refuse food, be unable to sleep, and feel sorry for himself. Later, his thinking shifts from looking back on life to looking forward to death. He may appear to be more cooperative but actually be more withdrawn. He may say little, sigh often, and stare into space.

In time he reaches the last stage, which is one of acceptance. Depression leaves him and he becomes calm about his fate, awaiting death with patience and dignity.

One important result of these studies has been the discovery that many patients want to talk about dying, to express their feelings, and to plan the rest of their lives. Talking and expressing feelings helps them through the four stages that precede acceptance of death. And talking may help the family to adjust their lives to the loss.

Geriatric patients usually accept death more willingly than younger adults. Death may even seem attractive to those who have lost many family members and friends or whose life-style has been changed by disability, pain, and limited income. Many older people have been threatened by death several times and so have experienced the five emotional stages of dying. Some have more fear of continued life than of dying.

In fact, the right to die has become an important issue among older people. Legal forms are now available for patients to sign. These forms request that, in the event of extreme conditions, no special efforts be made to prolong the signer's life.

The dying patient is often in physical distress and frightened. He may be extremely restless, gasping for breath, and disoriented. He may appear comatose or unconscious.

Even when he appears to be disoriented or unconscious, he may in fact have increased awareness of light, sounds, movements near him, touch, smell, and other sensory stimulants.

Every effort must be made to reduce irritating conditions and provide a comfortable, reassuring situation.

Care of a Dying Patient

Comfort the patient by staying with him as much as possible. Be very careful of conversation with the patient and others.

Do not say anything that may cause the patient mental distress.

Keep the room light and aired. Try to prevent any objectionable odors by keeping the patient as clean as possible.

Keep the patient warm, but make the top bedding light in weight and tuck it over a footboard to free the feet.

Give special mouth care, every hour, to keep the mouth moist. A thin application of oil over the lips prevents dryness.

Handle the patient very gently but change his position often. Placing the patient on his side helps mucus drain from the mouth or nose.

Check urinary output and be sure the patient does not have a full bladder to distress him. The doctor may do a catheterization if the bladder is full.

After-Death Care

Certain necessary attentions must be given a body soon after death to keep it as natural-looking as possible. These are done in any situation because the body stiffens as heat leaves it. Once hardened, body parts to do not move.

The body is laid flat on the back with one pillow under the head.

The eyes are closed.

Any dentures or other artificial parts, such as an eye, are placed in position on the body.

The body is cleaned.

The hands are folded on the chest.

17

Defective Vision and Hearing

Blindness

The legal definition of blindness is that while wearing prescription glasses, one is able to see only at 20 feet what the normal eye sees at 200 feet.

Although there are about 350,000 legally blind persons in the United States, the National Society for the Prevention of Blindness estimates that at least half of all cases could have been prevented or cured with present knowledge and equipment.

Today there are numerous organizations that help the legally blind. This help includes training in self-care, job training, job placement, and special educational and recreational methods that make it possible for blind children to attend the same schools as sighted children. The Library of Congress, in Washington, D.C., lends recordings and machines without charge to the blind.

Failing Vision

Particularly among older patients can be found those who are blind. Most of these, however, are not blind as a result of aging and, therefore, have had special training in adapting to their handicap. More common among the aged are those with poor or failing vision.

It is necessary only to close your eyes for a few minutes and attempt to carry on your everyday life in order to experience the confusion that a person with poor vision feels. The aged patient feels even more so. He is afraid of falling or otherwise hurting himself, afraid of being cut off from the normal life of people who can see, and afraid of losing his independence. All of these fears can be calmed.

Special Safety Measures

Remove unnecessary furniture from his room.

Remove throw rugs and anything else that may cause the patient to trip.

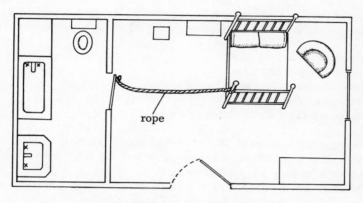

*Use a rope guide from bed to bathroom
for a patient with poor vision.*

Do not wax floors.

Arrange the furniture to suit his needs and to provide clear pathways to the bathroom and door. Use a guide rope to these areas if necessary.

Remove fragile glass objects that can shatter.

Have the room well lighted.

Block stairs and other dangerous areas.

If he enters a strange room, describe the room and its contents to him. If he is able, take him around the room so that he can touch the contents and orient himself.

Never leave a person with poor vision in the direct path of an obstacle. EXAMPLE: Never leave a patient facing a wheelchair or a wall.

When helping the person to a seat, put his hand on the arm or back of the chair. If this is impossible, walk up to the chair with him so that he is facing it. Tell him the location of the chair.

See that the person dresses in neat, becoming clothes, that his hair is trimmed and combed, and that his whiskers are shaved. Encourage a woman to use makeup and wear jewelry.

Marking Belongings

The belongings of a geriatric person with failing vision, but who is otherwise able, should be marked so that he can identify them by touch. This allows the patient to perform a maximum of self-care. A simple marking system can be taught and the patient encouraged to help in the marking. The patient should be able to identify

which items belong to him;
one item from another;
the front from the back of a garment;
one color from another;
two of a pair, such as gloves or socks.

When a patient must share storage space, such as a medicine cabinet, his toilet items can be identified by a rubber band or adhesive-tape strip put around them.

Different-sized containers help him identify one product from another. Color markings help him distinguish one garment from another.

Sew-on or iron-on tape in the center back of collars and waistbands allows him to tell front from back.

Sewing thread knots on the tape can be used to identify color. EXAMPLE: One knot for blue, two knots for brown.

Shoes can be marked for color by putting tape strips on the underarch. EXAMPLE: One strip for blue, two strips for brown.

When numbers of knots and tapes are used for colors, the same number should stand for the same color, regardless of marking material. EXAMPLE: One should always be blue and two always brown, regardless of whether the marking material is tape or knots.

Two socks or gloves can easily be kept mated if they are pinned together with a safety pin when the patient removes them. They can be washed, dried, and stored while pinned, and unpinned only when the patient is wearing them. (Use brass safety pins to prevent rusting.)

Arranging Closets

Hang all clothing of one kind together and always in the same place. EXAMPLE: Hang all long coats on the far right of a closet and all jackets on the near right.

Hang clothing according to frequency of use. EXAMPLE: The everyday coat should be first in the coat group, with the raincoat next and the dress coat last.

If plastic clothing bags are used, mark each one, in the same place near the zipper pull, with short strips of plastic tape to indicate its contents. EXAMPLE: One strip for dresses, two strips for coats, three strips for slacks.

Keep shoes together in pairs in boxes or a door shoebag. Boxes can be marked with plastic tape strips to identify the shoes. EXAMPLE: One strip for high heels, two strips for low heels. If a bag is used, keep pairs together in rows. EXAMPLE: First row, low heels; second row, high heels.

Arranging Drawers

Use boxes without covers as drawer dividers and put items of a kind into one box. For example, in all average dresser drawers, two shirt laundry boxes can provide three space divisions. Put shirts with front openings in one box, collarless slipover shirts in the other box, and turtlenecks in the space between them.

In shallow drawers, plastic egg cartons make good dividers for small objects.

Feeding the Patient

Unless the patient is too ill to do so, he should feed himself. He can manage very well if you

protect his clothing with a bib or napkin;
be sure he is in a comfortable eating position and that his tray or table setting is easy to reach;
set his tray with as few dishes and as little equipment as possible;
describe to him the location of every article on the tray and exactly what food or drink each dish or cup contains.

When describing a plate containing several kinds of food, have the patient imagine the plate as the face of a clock. Then describe the food in relationship to the clock. Say, "You have sliced carrots at eleven o'clock, mashed potatoes at three o'clock, and chopped steak at six o'clock." Meat is always positioned at six o'clock. With this image, the blind person has no difficulty in locating and selecting what he chooses to eat.

Prepare his food before he begins. Put sugar and milk on his cereal if he wants them. Butter his bread and cut his meat if he cannot manage otherwise.

Let him taste the food, then ask if he would like additional salt or pepper, and so forth.

Have cups or glasses only three-quarters full. Use plastic rather than china or glass.

Put straws in liquids.

Do not serve liquids that are very hot. Warn him of hot dishes or foods.

Try to avoid foods that are difficult for even the sighted to eat, such as peas, or prepare them in such a way as to make them manageable. EXAMPLE: Serve peas as pea soup or mix the peas with mashed potatoes.

If you must feed the patient, sit down beside him. Relax and make pleasant conversation or he will sense your anxiety and become nervous. Offer small bites. Tell the patient which food is in each bite, whether the bite is on a fork or a spoon, and whether that bite is hot or cold. If he is very ill or deaf, touch his cheek to signal that the spoon is ready.

Special Social Manners

See that the person with failing vision is included in groups that watch television or movies, plays, and sporting events. He is as interested in life and social contact as is a person who sees well.

Always address a blind person or one with failing vision directly and not through another person. EXAMPLE: Don't say, "Does he take tea or coffee?" Say, "Will you have coffee or tea, Bob?"

Always identify yourself before talking to the person with poor vision. Unless he knows you extremely well, he cannot identify you by your voice.

Always let the person know when you are leaving him so that he doesn't continue talking after you have gone. EXAMPLE: Say, "I have to leave you now, Bob."

When walking with a person who has poor vision, let him take your arm rather than your taking his. He can better balance himself and sense your moves if he holds onto you. If the way is too narrow to walk arm in arm, you go first, extending your arm behind you to take hold of his hand. While you walk single file, talk to him, describing anything in the way so that he is prepared for your movements. EXAMPLE: Say, "There's a table in our way just ahead. I'm going to move left to go around it."

Visual Aids

Most geriatric patients wear eyeglasses and are very dependent on them. In addition to eyeglasses, they may use hand-held or stand magnifying glasses. Large-print books and newspapers are also available.

Care of Eyeglasses

Check eyeglasses daily. They should be free of smudges, dust, and spots on the lenses. If you are cleaning lenses with a special eyeglass cleaning product, read the instructions on the label and follow them. Know if the lenses are glass or plastic. Never use polishing paper on plastic lenses.

The eyeglasses should sit straight and snug on the bridge of the nose. If hinges or earpieces are loose, the glasses can slip forward or be seated crooked, distorting vision. If earpieces are very loose, glasses may fall off when the patient looks down.

The glasses should not pinch, put pressure on, rub, or redden any part of the patient's nose or ears. If any of these things occurs, the glasses may be adjusted by a specialist and skin care given to the affected area.

Eyeglasses should always be stored in a protective pouch to prevent scratching or breaking. Never lay an eyeglass lens down on a hard surface.

Eyeglasses should always be kept in the same safe place within the patient's easy reach.

They should never be worn by anyone except the person to whom they were fitted.

Failing Hearing

Failing hearing may be caused by
blockage of the outer part of the ear canal;
accumulation of wax in the outer ear canal;
skin infection in the canal;
infection in the middle ear;
infection spreading to the bone around the ear;
a ruptured eardrum;
deposits on the bones of the middle ear;
nerve loss.

Only a doctor and sometimes only an ENT specialist (ear, nose, and throat doctor) can determine the cause of loss of hearing and treat it successfully.

Care of a Hearing Aid

Keep a hearing aid away from radiators, hair dryers, or other sources of high temperature. Heat deteriorates batteries and can damage an amplifier.

Keep it away from damp places. If the patient perspires a great deal, use silica gel (available from a hearing aid center). Place the aid and the gel in a plastic bag overnight. The aid will be dry in the morning.

Keep several spare batteries on hand. However, since batteries lose strength through aging, buy only a few at a time.

Wrap batteries in plastic if you carry them in a bag with other objects. The plastic will prevent their accidental contact with metal.

To lengthen the life of batteries, remove them from the aid during the night.

Keep battery contacts clean. Poor contacts cause power loss and a "sizzling" noise. If battery contacts should become eroded, take them to your dealer and let him clean them.

A defective aid drains a battery. If a battery loses power rapidly, have your dealer check the aid.

Unless the battery has a manufacturer's label that states that the battery can be recharged, don't do it.

Clean a clogged ear mold opening with a toothpick or pipe cleaner. From time to time, detach the mold and wash it with soapy water or with a special cleaning fluid obtainable from your dealer. A single drop of fluid can block sound and damage an aid. Alcohol should not be used to clean the ear mold because it dries the plastic. Solutions containing carbon tetrachloride should never be used.

Avoid twisting the cord or bending the tubing of an aid. Every so often, check the tubing or the cord for signs of wear.

Avoid dropping the aid or knocking it against hard objects.

Always turn the switch to the off position before taking off the aid. If the switch is left on, the batteries will run down.

Hair spray damages an aid. Don't use hair spray while wearing an aid.

Never try to repair a hearing aid yourself. Have it serviced by an expert.

Special Social Manners

Always face the person and look directly at him regardless of who is speaking.

Don't make noises, such as shuffling your feet, coughing, or clapping your hands, when conversing with him.

Keep room background noises to a minimum. EXAMPLE: Close a window on a noisy street or turn off a television before conversing with the person.

Listen to him attentively. Many people with hearing loss also suffer some speech difficulty.

Never shout, but do speak slowly and distinctly.

If he has a hearing aid, see that he uses it during conversation.

See that he always has a pad and pencil within easy reach so that he can write or read if he fails to communicate through speech or hearing.

Special Protection

Hearing can be affected by head colds, wind, and dust. The person with hearing loss should be protected from these.

18

Diabetes

Diabetes is a disease resulting from the body's inability to make enough insulin, a glandular secretion that controls the body's ability to utilize sugar. Insulin is produced in the pancreas. Without sufficient insulin, too much sugar stays in the blood and spills over into the urine.

To correct this imbalance the person's diet must be controlled to limit sugar intake, and in most instances insulin must be given, by injection or orally. The amount of insulin must balance the amounts and kinds of food the patient eats.

The doctor orders the following special care:

urine tests for sugar and acetone at exact times
a special diet
insulin to be given in exact doses at exact times
skin care

Urine Testing

A Clinitest or Testape urine testing package can be purchased at any drugstore.

Keep testing equipment together on a tray. Post the Clinitest or Testape chart on a nearby wall or inside a medicine cabinet door.

To Test for Sugar with Clinitest

Collect a fresh specimen from the patient at each of the times the doctor has ordered.

Take the urine to the bathroom.

Use a medicine dropper to transfer five drops of urine into a test tube.

Rinse the dropper and transfer ten drops of water into the same test tube.

Drop one tablet of Clinitest into the test tube. (Do not handle tablets; pour one tablet into the bottle cap and then into the test tube.)

Watch the reaction until fifteen seconds after the reaction stops.

Shake the test tube gently.

Hold the test tube near the Clinitest chart and compare the colors.

If the result is negative, mark this on a record sheet.

If the result is positive, mark the exact reading on a record sheet. Report the readings to the doctor at every visit.

To Test for Acetone with Acetest

Put an Acetest tablet on a dry white paper.

Use a medicine dropper to place one or two drops of urine on the tablet.

Wait sixty seconds and compare the color of the tablet with the Acetest color chart.

Mark the exact reading on the record sheet and report the reading (if positive) to the doctor.

To Test for Sugar with Testape

Another means of testing urine for sugar content is Testape. It is simple to use and is packaged in a small plastic container that is convenient to carry.

Collect urine in a clean container.

Check the expiration date on the Testape container; do not use tape with an expired date.

See that your hands are clean and dry.

Lift the lid of the container. Pull out about one and a half inches of tape. Continue to hold the tape straight out while closing the lid. After closing the lid, jerk the tape to release it from the container.

Pinch one end of the tape between your thumb and forefinger

and quickly dip the other end into the urine; remove tape immediately.

Continue to hold tape for one minute to allow for complete color development.

Match tape against color chart on Testape container.

If tape color reads +++, wait an additional half minute (thirty seconds) to see if there are further color changes. Compare tape and color chart again.

If the tests for sugar and acetone are strongly positive, the doctor may order extra insulin to be given before the next meal. He may change the patient's diet.

Diet

The doctor provides the patient with a special diet and instructs the patient on using it. The patient is allowed to select, from specific listings of foods and exact proportions, the menu for each of his meals. Only those foods and portions are permitted. *The patient must not eat other foods or amounts. No* sugar is allowed —

no sugar for table or tray use
no sugar-sweetened canned fruit
no sugar-sweetened gelatins, puddings, or ice creams
no sugar-sweetened pies, cakes, cookies, or candy
no sugar-sweetened soft drinks
no alcoholic drinks (Alcohol has a high sugar content.)
no oranges or other very sweet fruits unless specifically ordered

Saccharin may be used as a sugar substitute.

The patient must eat all the food prepared for his meal. If everything is not eaten, a description of what he left must be reported. EXAMPLE: The patient refused his entire serving of meat. He ate his vegetables and fruit but left half his bread and butter. A substitute meal may be necessary to balance his food intake with his insulin intake.

Insulin

Insulin must be given exactly as ordered to balance the patient's intake of food.

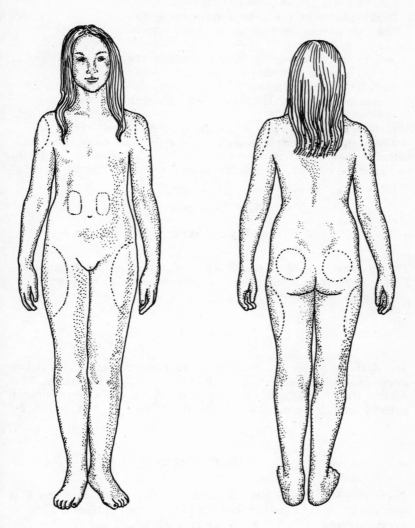

How insulin injection sites should be rotated

Insulin for injection must be kept in the refrigerator.
Oral insulin need not be kept in the refrigerator.
The patient must be watched for symptoms of

insulin shock (too much insulin): nervousness; cool, clammy
    skin; hunger; fainting;
diabetic coma (too much sugar): fruity odor to breath; fruity
    odor to urine; dry, hot skin; snorting breathing; coma.

If these symptoms appear, a doctor must be called at once.

The diabetic patient who goes out alone should wear an identification bracelet or carry a card that states, I AM A DIABETIC. Then, in the event of coma or shock, correct treatment can be given at once.

Eye Care

The diabetic should have his eyes examined every six months. Proper and prompt treatment can prevent or delay blindness.

Positioning

The diabetic patient is more prone to pressure sores, and if one develops, it is less likely to heal than in a nondiabetic patient. This patient therefore should have frequent checks on body alignment, activity, and skin condition. He should change position frequently.

Skin Care

Every diabetic should have a routine of skin inspection and care that eliminates the possibility of infection from cuts, scratches, or pressure sores.

His fingernails and toenails should be trimmed by a doctor, podiatrist, or other specially trained person. Hangnails should not be allowed to develop.

He should never wear clothing that binds, cuts, scratches, or irritates the skin. He should never wear shoes that pinch or rub.

He should use a soft toothbrush and also use mouthwash frequently.

Special Considerations for Older Patients

Reports on blood tests for detection of diabetes should be part of every checkup of a geriatric patient. Many patients develop the disease in later life, although such cases are often mild and can be controlled by diet alone or by diet and daily oral medication.

Diabetes can be very dangerous for the geriatric patient, however. Not only is he subject to the problems of the disease, but diabetes also complicates many other common diseases of aging. The diabetic patient with varicose veins who develops varicose ulcers, for example, is less likely to respond to treatment than is the nondiabetic patient. Diabetes increases susceptibility to any infection and lengthens any healing process in the patient. Gangrene and the necessity for amputation can develop from a pin scratch or any improperly trimmed toenail.

Amputation means surgical removal of a part of the body, such as a finger, arm, foot, or leg. With advancing age, blood circulation in the feet and legs becomes less and less efficient. As a result, infections there take longer to heal. When diabetes is also present, an infection can quickly spread through the foot or leg until gangrene develops. (Gangrene is the death of tissue from infection and inadequate blood circulation.) When this occurs, the affected part must be amputated to prevent the gangrene from spreading.

19

Fracture

A *simple* fracture is a break in the bone, but the bone does not pierce the skin.

A *compound* fracture is a break in a bone and the bone does pierce the skin.

First Aid

First aid for a fracture involves treatment for shock and the application of a splint to the affected body part. No effort should be made to undress, to pull on, or otherwise to adjust the fractured part. The splint helps prevent movement in the broken part until the patient can be treated by a doctor.

Equipment
blankets or other warm coverings
four or more strong cloth strips
a splint: any firm, straight, lightweight object that is about the
    length of the broken part
padding for the broken part

Reassure the patient.
Leave the patient where he has fallen or help him to lie down.
Place the patient flat on his back. Use care in extending the broken part.
Loosen any tight clothing.

Use the blankets to cover all of the patient's body except the affected part.

Put padding around the part.

Lay the splint beside the part so that the fracture is in the center of the splint.

Without tying, gently arrange all the cloth strips in position around the affected part and the splint so that the ends of the ties are on the outside of the splint.

Keeping the tension steady but not overly tight, knot the ties securely, tying them in the order of placement, and positioning the knots against the splint.

Treatment of a Fracture

A doctor treats a fracture by *reduction*. This means that he pulls and adjusts the bone edges until they are in their normal position.

If the break is simple, the doctor may do a *closed reduction,* one that does not require surgery.

If the break is compound, the doctor may do an *open reduction,* one that requires surgery.

Sometimes a doctor performs surgery on either a simple or a compound fracture in order to insert a metal pin, nail, plate, or screw into the bone to brace the break. This is called *internal fixation*. It is often used on geriatric patients because it allows more body motion than an external cast and, therefore, helps prevent health complications.

After reduction of the fracture, the doctor maintains correct positioning by applying a cast or traction to the broken part.

A *cast* is a hard covering molded to fit a body part so that the part maintains a fixed position.

Traction is the use of pulling force to correct and maintain normal positioning.

Application of a Cast

After reducing a fracture, the doctor covers all the body part to be contained by the cast with soft cotton stockinette. He then wets plaster gauze roll and applies it over the stockinette to build a thick shell. This hardens as it dries and braces and protects the break during healing.

Care of a Patient with a Cast

A cast takes a long time to dry and may still be damp when the patient is put to bed.

Use a bedboard to make the mattress firm.

Protect bedding by using a plastic mattress cover or a plastic drawsheet under the cast area.

Use only the palms of your hands to handle a damp cast. Fingers can cause pressure indentations in the cast.

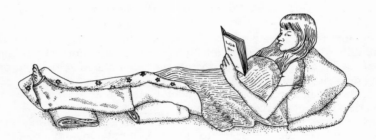

Allowing exposed cast to dry. Note: Folded towels under knee and heel; other leg covered by one baby blanket, torso by another.

Use small pillows under the curves of the cast to prevent the cast from cracking or changing shape.

Cover all the body except that in the cast with a sheet or cotton blanket. Leave the cast exposed to dry.

Turn the patient often to ensure even drying of the cast and to prevent skin pressure points.

Cover the parts of the cast that may be soiled by urine or feces with disposable plastic-backed padding.

Watch the skin around the cast and the fingers or toes for changes in color to very white or blue.

Watch also for swelling. Report such signs to the doctor at once.

Also report at once if the patient complains of numbness, pain, or tingling in the area covered by the cast.

An arm or a leg in a cast should be elevated to lessen swelling.

After the cast is dry, use self-adhering foam padding that is cut to size to pad pressure points made by the cast.

Traction

Traction is the use of sustained pulling force to correct and maintain body positioning. Traction can be applied in several ways:

by weights
by elastic
by special clothing
by skeletal bracing

Weight traction is applied by attaching one end of a rope to the extremity of the affected body part and stringing the other end over a pulley and weighting it. The poundage of the weights for each traction is specified by the doctor. Only people with special training can apply weight traction.

In elastic traction, an elastic appliance causes pull on the affected part.

Special clothing that braces and limits movement is usually made of combinations of leather, metal, plastic, and strong cloth. Surgical collars and corsets are examples of special traction clothing.

In skeletal traction, a doctor performs surgery to attach pins, wires, or tongs directly onto the bone.

Care of the Patient in Traction

Special skin care is necessary to prevent skin breakdown at pressure areas.

The patient's position must be changed on a regular schedule.

The doctor may order an overhead trapeze so that the bed patient can use it to lift himself when changing position. The patient should be taught and frequently reminded to pull straight on the bar when lifting himself. By doing so, he does not disturb the traction.

Both the patient and the traction equipment should be checked by all the people caring for the patient whenever they are approaching the bed.

See that the traction weights always hang free. (They should never be allowed to rest on a chair, the floor, or part of the bed.)

See that the patient has not slipped down in the bed. If he has, reposition him.

See that the patient is positioned so that nothing interferes with the traction.

When making the bed of a patient in traction, start making it on the patient's affected side. This disturbs the traction less.

If the patient complains of feeling chilled or if the affected part feels cold to your touch, cover the part in traction with a baby blanket or other lightweight covering.

Caring for the Elderly Fracture Patient

Aging makes people more accident prone. Diseases waste the body. Muscles lose tone. Eyesight, hearing, and touch sensitivity become less acute and lessen the person's ability to recognize danger. Slower reflexes reduce the ability to withdraw from danger. Mental confusion often interferes with an understanding of danger. Older people bump against objects, trip, slip, and fall more frequently than do younger adults. Since bones tend to grow brittle with age, a hard bump or a minor fall can cause a fracture.

The best geriatric fracture care, therefore, is preventive. All older people should be protected against the possibility of injury. Safety devices and techniques should be used in every aspect of geriatric care.

When a fracture does occur, the older patient does not heal quickly, and shock from the injury can disturb his health in many dangerous ways. Mental confusion, digestive upset, incontinence, bowel impaction, skin breakdown, pneumonia, pain, and stiffness are frequent complications of fractures in geriatric patients.

Every effort must be made to prevent these conditions and to treat any accident or complication immediately. Observe the fracture patient with special care, report and discuss with the doctor any changes in the patient's condition, and give emotional support as well as physical attention. In addition to other special nursing care, a geriatric fracture patient should receive the following as a routine:

intensive skin care
a change in position every two hours
careful supervision of fluid and food intake
careful bowel and bladder control

20

Heart and Lung Disease

The Cardiovascular Blood Vessel System

The heart is a muscular organ. Blood, filled with carbon dioxide and other wastes from all the cells of the body, enters the heart from the system of veins.

Contractions of the heart muscle send this blood to the lungs to be purified of carbon dioxide and wastes, and to take in oxygen.

The oxygenated blood returns to the heart and is pumped through the system of arteries to feed and give oxygen to all cells of the body.

The Respiratory System

Air, breathed in through the nose and mouth, passes along the trachea, or windpipe, past the larynx, or voice box, into the bronchial tubes, or main air tubes of the lungs. Many smaller tubes branch off the bronchial tubes, and those tubes branch until much of the lung is filled with tiny air passages. Most of the remaining lung is filled with tiny blood vessels.

Fresh air, containing oxygen, is inhaled into the lungs and exchanged for one of the body's waste products, carbon dioxide, which is exhaled. The carbon dioxide is carried by the blood system to the lungs from all body cells.

The act of breathing is controlled by a large muscle that lies under the lungs. This muscle is the diaphragm. The expansion of the diaphragm causes a sucking in of air, or inhalation. The contraction of the diaphragm squeezes air from the lungs. This is called exhalation.

Inhalation is also called inspiration; exhalation is also called expiration. One act of inspiration and expiration is called respiration.

Because the heart and lungs are connected and dependent on each other, disease of one usually causes distress in the other.

Aging in particular causes changes in the heart and blood vessels that result in disease. Most elderly patients eventually suffer from some chronic form of this disease. Some common forms of heart and blood vessel disease are

hypertension, or high blood pressure;
arteriosclerosis, or hardening of the arteries;
coronary thrombosis, or heart attack;
aneurysm, or weakening of an arterial wall;
heart failure.

There are many kinds of heart diseases, so care of a cardiac patient always depends on three things:

the diagnosis
the severity of the illness
the orders of the individual doctor

However, certain forms of treatment are accepted by most doctors as being helpful to the very ill heart patient. They include rest, positioning, oxygen, and a special diet. All of these are meant to place the least strain on a sick heart.

Determination of heart disease is made by the doctor after physical examination, blood tests, blood pressure readings, and an electrocardiogram.

Electrocardiogram (EKG or ECG)

An EKG machine is an electric box (usually mounted on a wheeled table) with wires attached to it that are glued to the skin of the patient's chest, arms, and legs. A trained person operates a panel on the box to measure the patient's heart activity and to trace it on graph paper. The tracing is then studied for differences from normal tracings.

Acute Symptoms

Patients without previous signs of heart or blood vessel disease sometimes develop acute symptoms, and patients with chronic disease sometimes have acute attacks. Acute symptoms include severe chest pain, difficulty in breathing, blue color to skin, irregular pulse, anxiety, and dizziness. Whenever acute symptoms develop, the patient requires special care. If he is very ill, he may be moved to a hospital or coronary care unit where a cardiac monitor can be used. A coronary care unit is a special area provided with machines and personnel to observe and give intensive care to heart patients.

Care of a Patient with Acute Symptoms

CARDIAC MONITOR

A cardiac monitor is an electric machine that can be attached by wire to the patient's skin. The machine records a continuous pattern of the patient's heart activity and projects it on a TV-like screen. A trained observer can read the patient's immediate condition by a glance at the screen.

Other aspects of patient care for acute symptoms may include

rest;
positioning;
oxygen;
special diet;
intravenous feedings to regulate the sodium and potassium balance of the blood.

REST

Physical Rest. The doctor orders complete bed rest at first and then gradual activity.

He orders mild laxatives to keep the patient's bowels open so that there is no danger of an attack through straining to expel a hard stool. Be alert for any sign of constipation and report it at once.

Move the patient as gently as possible. (Passive exercises may be ordered.)

Anticipate the patient's needs so he does not have to speak.

Provide a pleasant, airy, comfortable room with no bright lights.

Keep the room as free of noise as possible.

Be pleasant and cheerful but not talkative.

Give special care to the patient's skin to prevent breakdown.

Mental Rest. At first the patient is not allowed to read, watch television, or listen to the radio.

A telephone should be removed from the room.

He should be assured about his business or his concern for his family.

Emotional Rest. Visiting is allowed only as the doctor orders and is usually restricted to family at first. Visits should be short, a few minutes at a time, and talking limited. Visitors must be warned not to upset the patient by weeping or telling him about problems.

End a visit at any small sign of distress or fatigue on the part of the patient.

POSITIONING IN BED

The body is placed in a position that makes it easiest for the patient to breath. The patient's head and chest are elevated. Supports, such as pillows, are put under his knees and forearms. Sometimes he is positioned sitting and bent forward in the bed with his arms resting on an overbed table that has been padded with pillows.

OXYGEN (O_2)

Be sure all safety rules are carried out.

Be sure the liter reading is correct.

Check the amount in the tank often.

Reorder tanks as needed.

Watch and report the patient's reaction to oxygen.

SPECIAL DIET

Follow the doctor's orders exactly. He may order any combination of the following diets: soft, low-salt, low-cholesterol, or low-calorie, as well as other specific requirements.

If a patient is in a nursing facility, the diet is prepared by the diet kitchen. If the patient is at home, you can easily prepare his food by using a diet sheet provided by the doctor.

Chronic Symptoms

Patients with chronic heart and blood vessel disease may tire easily, be short of breath, or have irregular breathing, coughing, and wheezing. They may have periods of dizziness, swelling of the ankles and legs, and periods of pain in the chest, neck, and left arm. They may be very pale or very red or have bluish lips and fingernails.

Care of a Patient with Chronic Symptoms

Most doctors agree that patients with chronic heart disease should be as physically active as possible. Walking and mild exercise are desirable. The patient should avoid emotional stress, mental pressures, and overtiring himself.

He may be more comfortable resting in a sitting position than lying in bed. A large, comfortable armchair with a footrest should be provided.

Most doctors agree that excess weight contributes to heart and blood vessel problems. The patient therefore should have a diet that will keep him thin.

Tight clothing should never be worn.

He should have frequent reevaluations.

He should have the right medication for his condition.

Medications Often Used in Heart Disease

Diuretics

This medication draws edema (unwanted fluid) from the patient's tissues. As a result, the patient may urinate more frequently. Any patient who is taking a diuretic should be on measured intake and output.

Nitroglycerine

This medicine dilates the blood vessels when a tablet is placed under the tongue. The medicine must be used very quickly by certain patients when they feel approaching distress. This drug is always kept within the patient's ready reach; at night it should be placed on a table at his bedside and during the day in a handy pocket of his clothing. The tablet container should be placed in the same locations every night and day.

Oxygen

Sometimes a doctor allows a patient to operate an oxygen tank that is kept at his bedside but used only when he feels the need for it. An oxygen mask is the usual form of delivery. When oxygen is used in this way, check the tank frequently to see that safety precautions are observed (see page 256).

Respiratory Disease

Common Respiratory Diseases

Emphysema. A loss of function in the lungs as a result of air pollution, smoking and aging. Breathing is difficult.

Tuberculosis (TB). An infectious disease caused by a specific organism. It responds well to modern medication.

Lung Cancer. A growth in the lung often caused by irritation from cigarette smoking.

Any patient with respiratory problems is more apt to get respiratory infections, such as colds, flus, and pneumonias, than is the average person. Preventive care must be taken.

Many patients have deep coughs that produce sputum. Any such patient should always have at hand a clean disposable container, with a cover, into which he can spit. Containers should be changed daily and more often if necessary. Isolation technique should be used when disposing of containers containing infectious material.

Patients with respiratory problems may receive inhalation therapy to stimulate breathing. They may be taught special breathing and coughing techniques. Postural drainage and steam inhalations may be ordered.

They may move slowly because rapid movements increase breathing difficulties. They may pant, wheeze, whistle, and have bluish or pale and moist skin. Chest movements are usually very noticeable. When in bed these patients should always have their heads elevated to make breathing easier.

Postural Drainage

The doctor sometimes orders postural drainage for a patient with respiratory disease. The patient is positioned with his head and chest lower than his hips so that secretions can drain from his lungs into his mouth and he can spit them out.

Postural drainage can be done in a hospital-type bed with the patient jackknifed over a fully elevated headrest. Or drainage can be done with the patient lying across the bed with his head and shoulders lowered over the side. For the patient who is allowed out of bed, the following method is easy and comfortable.

GIVING POSTURAL DRAINAGE USING AN UPHOLSTERED ARMCHAIR

Equipment
    a large plastic sheet or newspapers
    a disposable bag
    a large disposable container
    tissues
    a low-backed upholstered armchair

Cover the chair seat, arms, and seat back with the plastic sheet or newspapers.

Place the disposable container in the center of the chair seat.

Help the patient to stand behind and to bend over the chair back, so that his elbows rest on the chair arms and his chest and head hang over the container.

Tell him to take deep breaths and to cough so that secretions will loosen and start to drain. Turning from side to side during the coughing and deep breathing helps get drainage from all lung areas.

Have him cover his mouth with tissues while coughing to prevent the spread of germs.

Place the disposable bag so that the patient can put used tissues in it directly after using them.

As secretions drain tell the patient to spit into the container on the chair seat.

Have the patient remain in this drainage position from five to fifteen minutes, depending on the doctor's orders and on how the patient responds to the treatment.

Watch the patient for signs of weakness, dizziness, or overtiring. Stop the treatment if this occurs.

Inhalation Therapy

Some conditions, such as heart diseases and emphysema, are treated with inhalation therapy upon a doctor's orders.

Inhalation means the process of drawing air or gas into the lungs. Tanked gases, such as oxygen and carbon dioxide, are used in inhalation therapy.

No one should give, regulate, or shut off inhalation equipment unless he is familiar with the specific order for the patient and with the administration of the specific gas ordered.

Giving Oxygen (O_2)

THE O_2 TANK

Tanked oxygen is tightly contained in heavy steel that prevents the gas from escaping. A special head with two valves regulates the flow of oxygen and the speed of the flow. When a doctor orders oxygen, he also orders the speed at which it is to be given. His order might read: O_2 at 6 liters per minute. A liter is the measuring unit of the O_2 flow.

Tanked O_2 can be given
  by oxygen tent;
  by nasal catheter;
  by nasal cannula;
  by nose and mouth mask.

The O_2 Tent. This is a light, movable tent made of clear plastic and attached to a special sparkproof motor-driven unit. The motor circulates and cools the air inside the tent. The usual rate of O_2 flow in a tent is 10 to 12 liters. A thermostat keeps the temperature within the tent at about 70° F. (21° C.). It is quite drafty inside the tent and the patient's head and shoulders should be protected by towels. The tent fits over the head of the bed so that the patient's head and chest are inside. The back and sides of the tent are tucked as far under the mattress as they will go.

The tent front is folded within a folded drawsheet and that sheet tucked in on each side of the bed so that no oxygen leaks out.

There are zippered openings on both sides of the tent through which patient care is given. These openings should be closed except when care is in progress.

When the bed is made, the tent is moved from one side of the bed to the other with the patient.

Nasal Catheter or Tube. A small catheter is inserted into the nose by either a doctor or a nurse and strapped with adhesive to the forehead. The catheter connects to larger tubing that connects to either a wall O_2 supply or a tank. The flow of O_2 is usually 4 to 6 liters per minute. The tubing should be pinned to the sheet near the head of the bed to prevent pull on the catheter.

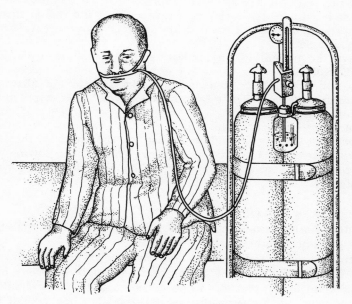

Patient using oxygen by himself by way of nasal cannula

Nasal Cannula. A nasal cannula for oxygen is made of plastic and is disposable. Two short tubes enter the patient's nostrils and are held in place by an adjustable strap that fits over the ears and under the chin. This is a very convenient method of administering O_2 and the patient is often able to use it himself without aid. The flow is usually 4 to 6 liters.

Mask. A mask fits tightly over the nose and mouth and is attached to the O_2 supply by tubing. The flow of O_2 is usually 8 liters.

SAFETY RULES

DANGER: When pure O_2 is given, chances of fire or explosion are great. Steps must be taken to avoid disaster. Safety rules must be followed.

Post NO SMOKING signs in any room where O_2 is used.

One sign is usually posted at the entrance and another on the O_2 tank.

See that the patient and his visitors are warned of the danger and cautioned against lighting matches.

Do not use ordinary electrical things in the area. These would include heating pads, stoves, razors, machines, and radios. Special sparkproofed equipment, such as the motor for an O_2 tent, is used when necessary.

Have the patient use a hand-rung dinner bell instead of an electric call bell.

Do not wear fabrics that cause sparks and do not allow the patient to wear them. These fabrics include wool, silk, rayon, nylon, and other synthetics.

Put cotton blankets on the bed.

The glass jar, or humidifier, must be kept filled with water to the measure marked on the glass. When O_2 is flowing, the water bubbles. Oxygen is very drying; bubbling it through water moistens it.

WATCHING AN O_2 TANK

Before starting a new tank, check the label on the tank to be sure it is O_2 and not another gas.

Temperature changes expand and contract oxygen. To allow for such changes the meter of a tank reads to 3,000, but the tank is considered full if it registers 2,000. At home, a new tank should be ordered when the meter on the one in use reads 1,000, or half full, for a delivery may take several days.

Oxygen tanks are very heavy, and because of this they are delivered strapped to special carriers. While in use, a tank should remain strapped on its carrier and care should be taken to prevent dropping it.

STARTING, OR CRACKING, AN O_2 TANK

A new tank must be "cracked" or opened and the "head," or part that consists of the meters, valves, and humidifier, fitted to it. This is done by trained personnel. For immediate use, the valve of the tank is opened until the capacity registers on the gauge. Then the liter regulator is opened and set at the desired reading. Both of these openings are right turns.

SHUTTING OFF AN O₂ TANK

First close the valve on the tank until the indicator on the meter drops to zero. Then allow any remaining oxygen to run out. (The water will stop bubbling and the liter gauge fall.) Then close the liter valve. Both of these are left turns.

Artificial Respiration

Artificial respiration is the forcing of the breathing process after breathing has stopped.

Mouth-to-mouth resuscitation is the form of artificial respiration that is most effective for emergency use. When properly given, it can save the life of a person whose heart is beating but whose breathing has stopped.

Breathing may stop from many causes such as drowning, electric shock, poisoning, chest injury, and suffocation. The absence of the rise and fall of the chest is a good indication that breathing has stopped. Whether or not you know the cause of respiratory failure, begin mouth-to-mouth resuscitation.

Artificial respiration must be started within minutes after breathing stops, otherwise death cannot be prevented. A doctor or emergency service should be called as soon as possible. If you must choose between calling the doctor and giving resuscitation, give resuscitation.

GIVING MOUTH-TO-MOUTH RESUSCITATION

Position the patient flat on his back.

Reach into his mouth and throat with your fingers and remove anything that might be clogging the passage.

Using both of your hands, tilt the patient's head back so that the jaw juts out (lift his chin with one hand, press his forehead with your other palm).

Maintaining this jutting jaw position, cover and seal the patient's open mouth with your mouth. Place your thumb and index finger at the end of the patient's nose.

Blow into the patient's mouth while pinching his nostrils shut.

Lift your mouth from the patient's and unclamp his nose. Take a breath and at the same time, press your other palm against the upper center of his abdomen.

Repeat about twenty times.

If you feel reluctant to place your mouth directly on the patient's, spread a handkerchief or other thin cloth over the patient's mouth before applying your own.

Respirator

A respirator is a machine that forces air into the lungs and causes deep breathing. It is often referred to by trade name. Both the Bird and the Bennet respirators are widely used, and reference to a Bird or a Bennet specifies its manufacturer. When both are available, check the trademark to identify each.

A respirator is ordered by a doctor when a patient's own breathing becomes impaired. Only a trained person should operate a respirator.

A respirator is used

to help stretch and tone respiratory muscles and lung tissues;
to help the patient cough up secretions without tiring;
to help deliver medication to deep areas of the lungs;
to help with the respirations of a patient with limited breathing ability;
to cause respirations in a patient who is completely unable to breathe by himself.

The respirator can be used in two ways: (1) the patient or an attendant can have control and can start and stop the machine as desired or (2) the machine can be set on automatic control.

Respirator air is delivered to the patient by means of either a mouthpiece or a mask. Whichever method is used, it is very important that no air leaks around the mouthpiece or mask.

If a mouthpiece is used, the patient is told to bite on it gently and to close his lips tightly around it; he should not breathe through his nose while the respirator is in use. Sometimes a nasal clamp is used to prevent breathing through the nose.

If a mask is used, the patient's face should be wiped free of skin oil before the mask is applied. This helps to prevent the mask from slipping.

After starting the respirator, check all tube connections and the mouthpiece or mask for air leaks.

During use of the respirator, both the patient and the machine should be checked constantly. The patient should be checked for skin color changes, respiratory difficulty, and pulse change.

Until a patient becomes accustomed to a respirator, he may be frightened by it. If he is alert, he must be reassured. The operation of the machine should be explained to him, and he should control it whenever possible.

After he has become accustomed to it, he may become dependent on the machine and not make an effort to breathe. He may panic if the respirator is taken away. This patient requires encouragement to breathe on his own. He may feel reassured if the respirator is left by his bedside, ready for use if necessary.

Steam Inhalation

The doctor may order steam inhalation for the patient with respiratory infection or disease. Breathing moist hot air often helps relieve lung congestion. Sometimes medicine is given through steam inhalation.

GIVING A STEAM INHALATION
Equipment
  an electric vaporizer
  medication (if ordered by the doctor)
  two bath towels
  water for the vaporizer
  a sputum cup
  tissues

Be sure you understand how your particular vaporizer operates. If in doubt read the instructions or ask someone who knows.

Fill the vaporizer water container to the level marked.

If medicine has been ordered, put the correct amount in the vaporizer medicine container.

Take the vaporizer to the bedside and position it near to and directed toward the patient. Be sure to put it where it cannot be a safety hazard, on the floor or on a table.

Plug in and turn on the vaporizer and wait until it begins to steam.

Cover the patient's head and hair with one towel. Put the other around his shoulders. The towels absorb some of the moisture.

A croup tent can be made by draping a cotton blanket over two unplugged lamp poles positioned on each side of the bedstead. A croup tent holds steam and so increases the concentration of vapor inhaled by the patient.

In an emergency, turn on the hot shower or tub faucet and allow the bathroom to become steamy. Have the patient sit in the bathroom until his breathing eases. Dry the patient well and change his clothes after the treatment.

21

Mental Disorders

Regardless of its cause, a mental disorder is always complex and peculiar to the individual because it includes all his life experiences, his health and family histories, and his social and economic background. The main cause of a mental disorder, however, is always either emotional or physical.

Emotional Disorders

Mental disorders of emotional origin are very common among patients and are often combined with physical causes. Loneliness, fears of the future, of death, of rejection by children, and frustrations over failing vision, hearing, or mobility can trigger mental disorder in a patient.

Of all these, perhaps loneliness is the worst. Scientists working with healthy animals produce mental disorders in them simply by isolating them from others of their kind. When isolation is added to physical disabilities, it is easy to imagine the unfortunate effect.

Mental disorders from emotional causes often respond very favorably if the patient receives loving, protective care and stimulating society.

Physical Causes

Many mental disorders of physical cause can affect both young and old. Some of these causes are infections, drugs, alcohol, head injury, brain tumor, and inadequate diet.

Two other disorders of physical cause occur only in older people. They are hardening of the head arteries (cerebral arteriosclerosis) and death of brain tissue from age (senile brain disease). These two diseases cause the destruction of brain cells and are known as chronic brain disease.

Once destroyed, brain cells cannot be restored. Brain damage is permanent, and a person can never learn, understand, remember, or manage a body function if the brain control center has been destroyed. If the speech area is destroyed, for example, the patient cannot speak words unless another area of his brain is trained to accept the function. Then he must relearn to speak, just as a child. He has no knowledge or memory of speech to help him.

Some older people have both forms of chronic brain disease. Although these patients should be maintained at the highest level of mental ability possible, they need special care as they become less and less able to function. Most eventually become irrational and incontinent, and require total care.

Symptoms

Whether originating from emotional or physical causes, all mental disorders cause changes in the personality of a person. Some signs of such changes include the following:

anxiety
confusion
depression
overactivity
underactivity
talkativeness
silence
angry outbursts
incontinence

weeping without cause
laughing without cause
talking to one's self
withdrawal from others
complaining or demanding behavior
forgetfulness

Caring for the Disturbed Patient at Home

See that the patient has whatever professional help he may require. This help is available through health centers, mental health centers, emergency room services, or private doctors.

Always treat the patient in as normal a manner as possible.

Allow the patient to do as much for himself and for others as he can.

Encourage but don't force him to do it.

Most disturbed patients are treated with drugs that help them to adjust to life. It is most important that they take such drugs in the right dosage and at the right times. It may be necessary to check the inside of the mouth to be sure that the patient has swallowed his tablet or capsule.

Include the patient in as many social situations as possible. At home, let him eat with others, watch TV with others, and the like. Take him outside to whatever activity and entertainments he can tolerate.

Observe the patient's physical and mental conditions and report changes.

See that the patient has food, water, and bowel and bladder control.

Do not react to the patient's actions. If the patient has an angry outburst, for example, do not become angry or scold him. Keep calm and be kind at all times.

Always talk to the patient when you are with him.

Touch the patient in a slow, gentle way whenever possible. Touch is especially important for patients with loss of hearing or vision.

Mental Disturbance in Children

Because all children show symptoms of emotional disturbance to degrees that would be abnormal in adolescents or adults, it is sometimes difficult to determine the boundary between health and overreaction.

Aggression relieves internal emotional conflicts by expressing them in hostile actions. The overly aggressive and hostile child shows a need to dominate in order to cover his need for dependency and protective care. Feelings of inferiority, resentment, inadequacy, and guilt motivate him to expose himself constantly to dangerous situations.

Anxiety is an unconscious fear that can often appear to be without cause. The cause lies in the child's inability to understand a threat to his security. If, for example, a baby is left alone for ten minutes, he has no way of knowing that the condition is temporary. He fears that he is being abandoned forever.

Anxiety can lead to phobia, or concentration of fears on a specific object or situation. The real threat is not the object of the phobia, but the child is able to relieve his anxiety by avoiding the phobia. Common phobias are fear of the dark, fear of an animal or all animals, fear of heights, fear of crowds, and fear of germs.

Anxiety can also lead to depression, which is a reduction in vitality and ability to function on both physical and mental levels. A depressed child is sometimes overactive and seems consumed with energy. He may lose his appetite, have frequent nightmares, and cry often.

A psychiatrist or therapist may use several forms of treatment to help a disturbed child. These include play therapy, group therapy, special schooling, change of environment, and specific medication.

Play Therapy

In play therapy a child is permitted to play with any article he wishes in a well-equipped playroom. A psychiatrist or therapist observes the child, encouraging him to talk and play fully. Through such contact the observer learns about a child's feelings, emotional reactions, and interests. He also learns about the child's relationships with himself, adults, his family, teachers, and playmates.

The therapist accepts the child just as he is and allows him to release tensions by expressing anger and being resistant, offensive, or submissive. There is no attempt by the therapist to change the child; change occurs through self-expression.

Group Therapy

In group therapy several children play together and express their problems in the presence of a therapist. The group members help each other by providing emotional support, acceptance, and a willingness to listen. Through such therapy a child learns to co-operate, share, and help others. He learns self-restraint and self-assertion.

22

Stroke

Age increases the chances of a person having a stroke, or cerebral vascular accident (CVA). The word *cerebral* refers to the brain, the word *vascular,* to the blood vessel system. Cerebral vascular accident therefore means an accident to the blood vessel system of the brain.

Normal nerve cells receive and interpret the messages of the senses (sight, hearing, smell, touch, and taste). Normal nerve cells also control movements. A CVA interferes with the blood supply to a part of the brain and, consequently, with the function of the nerve cells centered there.

Causes

Some of the many causes of a CVA are
   a clot forming in a blood vessel of the brain;
   a clot forming elsewhere in the body but carried by the blood to the brain;
   a torn blood vessel that allows bleeding into the brain;
   pressure on a blood vessel caused by a tumor or swelling;
   a spasm of a brain artery.

Prestroke Symptoms

Signs that may indicate approaching stroke are: severe headache, blurred vision, difficulty in speaking, dizziness or fainting, and numbness in a hand or a side of the face.

Understanding the Stroke Patient

Until a stroke occurs, the patient has the full use of his body. With the onset of a stroke, he loses consciousness, and when he recovers, he does not know what has happened to him. He is frustrated, frightened, and unaware of the existence of his affected side.

He may be unable to speak or to understand when someone speaks to him.

If approached, spoken to, or given directions by one standing on his affected side, he may not understand or respond.

He may have visual problems. For example, from a plate of food he may eat only that which lies within the visual range of his unaffected side.

He may have hemiplegia (be unable to move the arm and leg on the affected side).

The blood circulation on the affected side may be impaired.

He may have loss of sensation on the affected side.

He may be very forgetful and unable to concentrate.

He may tire easily.

His behavior may be inconsistent.

His balance while sitting and standing may be poor.

He may lose control of urine or bowels or both.

Hemiplegia

A CVA often causes hemiplegia, or the loss of ability to move and loss of feeling in one side of the body. The paralysis occurs on the opposite side of the brain from the affected part. For example, when a CVA occurs on the left side of the brain, the right side of the body is affected.

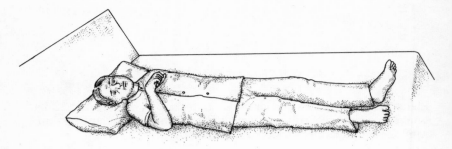

How body is affected by stroke

Under normal conditions, muscles that bend a body part are stronger than muscles that straighten a part. When stroke occurs, the muscles that straighten are weakened. The result is that the muscles that bend then pull the affected side.

One may observe the following responses:

The patient's head droops to the affected side.
The eyelid and mouth on the affected side may droop.
The arm is bent and hugs the chest.
Wrist, fingers, and thumb are bent.
The entire leg is extended and rotated outward.
The foot is on tiptoe and turned inward.
The entire body trunk tends to bend forward.

Stages

In the treatment of stroke, three progressive stages are recognized. Not all patients experience all three stages, however. Some may remain in the first stage; some progress to only the second stage. These stages are

flaccid — the affected side is weak and limp;
spastic — the affected side develops tense muscles;
recovery — the affected side returns to usefulness and is neither flaccid nor spastic.

Setting Up a Care Area

Arrange the unit furniture so that the patient's unaffected side is toward the bedside stand and open unit area.

See that the bed
   is a single or twin size;
   is waist high;
   has a firm mattress;
   has a bedboard;
   has a covered footboard;
   has a supply of towels, pillows, and blankets for positioning;
   has side rails.

See that the following are available for use:
   a washbasin
   soap in a soap dish
   washcloths and towels
   bedpan (and urinal if patient is male)
   emesis basin
   massage lotion
   box of tissues
   water pitcher
   plastic water glass
   bent paper straws or drinking tube

Vital Signs

The patient's blood pressure and temperature are taken often during the acute phase of a CVA. (The frequency depends on the doctor's instructions and the severity of the CVA.) The blood pressure readings are usually very unstable at first. The patient is kept on complete bed rest until the blood pressure stabilizes. It is not unusual for a stroke patient to have a fever during the acute signs of a CVA.

Stroke Positioning

Stroke positioning and ROM exercises are extremely important in the care of a patient with a CVA because they prevent wasting (atrophy) of muscles and further crippling of the affected side. They also enable the patient to recover maximal function.

General Rules for Stroke Positioning

Place the patient on a firm mattress.
Don't elevate the head or foot of the bed.
Always keep the head and spine in alignment.
Do not position the patient on his affected side.
Alternate limb positions between extensions and flexion.
Always keep the feet in neutral position.
Change the patient's position from back to good side, front, and then back every two hours.

Backlying Position

See that the spine and head are in a straight line.
Do not use a pillow under the head.

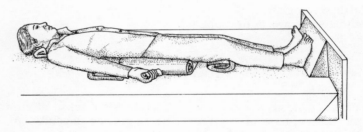

Correct back position in bed

Roll towels and fit them into the spaces under the neck, at the small of the back, under the knees, and in the affected hand.
Place the soles of the feet flat against an upright brace so that the feet cannot drop forward. Use a footboard or covered box as the brace.
Use a rolled blanket (trochanter roll), sandbags, or unopened food cans rolled in towels to brace the outside of the affected leg.

Side Position

Never turn the patient onto his affected side except for a few minutes, such as when making the bed.

Before turning the patient, always position the arm on the side to which the patient will turn. Raise that forearm beside the patient's head by rotating the shoulder. Cross the other arm over the chest.

After turning the patient, see that the spine and head are in a straight line.

Support the head with a pillow.

Support the affected arm with a pillow.

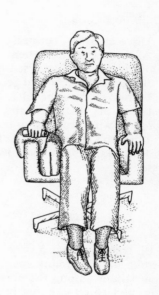

Sitting position. Note: One pillow under affected arm and another squeezed between chair side and affected leg.

Lift the top leg off the lower one and flex the knee.

Support the knee and leg with a pillow.

Frontlying (Prone) Position

Do not use a head pillow.

Remove the footboard.

Pull the mattress to the head of the bed.

Turn the patient onto his stomach.

Turn his head toward his affected side.

Move his body downward in the bed until his feet hang over the mattress edge in a neutral position. If it is impossible for the patient's feet to hang over the mattress, place a large pillow under his shins so that the knees are bent and the feet held in a neutral position.

Place a small pillow or folded towel under the patient's chest or lower part of the abdomen and hips.

Extend the affected arm upward toward the head of the bed or downward.

Put a rolled towel in the hand.

Chair Positioning

Use a chair with armrests.

After seating the patient, pull his buttocks forward a few inches. This gives him a better seating balance.

See that his body is in good alignment.

Stabilize his affected leg by wedging a pillow or rolled towel between his thigh and the arm of the chair. Support the affected forearm with a pillow so that his shoulders are even.

Put a roll in the patient's hand.

Encourage him to hold his head erect and tilted to the unaffected side.

Rehabilitation Through ADL

ADL training plays a very large part in the nursing care plan of the stroke patient. Many months of slow, continuous teamwork with the patient among the personnel of Physical Therapy, ADL Training, and Nursing departments and his family may be required in order to rehabilitate him.

Self-Help Moving, Turning, and Positioning by the Hemiplegic

MOVING FROM ONE SIDE OF THE BED TO THE OTHER

Lying on his back, the patient hooks his good foot under his affected knee and pulls the leg until the knee is bent and the affected foot rests flat on the mattress.

He then puts his unaffected leg in the same position and pushes on his good foot, lifting his hips and moving them in the desired direction.

He moves his head and shoulders by pushing or pulling on the side rail with his good hand.

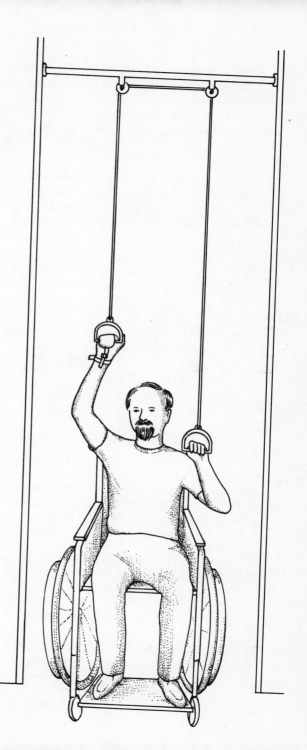

*Exercising affected arm
with pulley*

ROLLING OVER

The patient elevates both knees in the same manner as when he moves from one side of the bed to the other.

With his good hand, he pushes both knees in the direction of the turn and allows the knees to fall. This partly rolls his body.

He rolls the rest of his body by pushing or pulling on the side rail with his good hand.

SITTING UP IN BED (USING A BEDROPE)

A rope attached to the center of the foot of the bed can be used by the hemiplegic. Pulling on it with his good hand, he raises himself from a lying to a sitting position in bed.

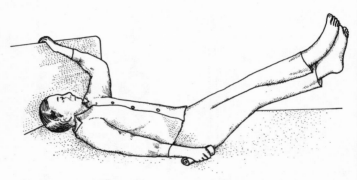

Exercising affected leg with good leg

MOVING TO A DANGLING POSITION (USING A BEDROPE)

The patient lies on his back in the center of the bed and uses his good hand to cross his affected arm over his abdomen.

He moves his legs to the side of the bed until his feet and ankles extend over the side.

He pulls on the bedrope with his good hand, raising himself to a sitting position. His legs automatically fall over the bedside.

Exercises

Specific passive and active exercises are ordered at different stages of hemiplegia. As the patient progresses, he is taught to use his unaffected side to exercise his affected side. You must be sure of which passive exercises you must do for the patient and which active exercises he should do by himself.

Skin Care

Because of changes in his blood circulation, incontinence, and the dead weight of his paralyzed side, the patient with a CVA is susceptible to pressure sores. Skin care should be given at every opportunity.

Bowel and Bladder Control

Most stroke patients have some urinary and bowel incontinence during the acute phases of illness. A patient may recover spontaneously or need one or more of the following: care for incontinence, Foley catheter drainage, condom drainage, enemas, suppositories, digital stimulation to remove feces, and retraining.

Bathing and Grooming

Bathing

The hemiplegic requires bed baths until he is allowed out of bed.

Once he is able to be up and about, he should have showers rather than baths because transferring him in and out of a bathtub is difficult and dangerous.

During a shower, he will need help washing his unaffected arm, both armpits, and other areas he cannot reach.

If no shower is available, the patient can be showered with a spray hose in the bathtub. He should sit in the tub or on a nonslip chair with a backrest.

ADL BATH AIDS

A long-handled bath sponge with a pocket for soap allows the patient to reach and soap nearly all his body.

A bath mitt with a pocket for soap is also useful. A hand brush with suction cups to stabilize it allows the patient to scrub his hand and nails on the unaffected side. This type of brush can also be used by the patient to scrub dentures.

Toilet products packaged in plastic spray containers are more easily managed and safer for the hemiplegic than are those in screw-top glass jars.

Shaving

An electric razor is easier and safer than a safety razor for the stroke patient to use.

Nail Care

A nail file or emery board taped to a tabletop allows the patient to file the nails of his unaffected hand.

Dressing the Hemiplegic Patient

Clothing should be oversized, fit loosely, and have easy closures in front or at the side. Wraparound or front-opening dresses with large buttons or Velcro fasteners are best. Short sleeves are easiest to manage. If sleeves are long, the wrist edges should be wide enough to admit the hand with ease. Half slips are easier than full slips for the female patient. Ready-tied bow ties are best for men. Button flies are easier for the patient to manage than zippers.

Forgetfulness often accompanies hemiplegia. The patient therefore may need step-by-step reminders in order to dress himself.

The affected side is always dressed first.

The unaffected side is always undressed first.

It is usually easiest to dress or undress the lower part of the body in bed.

If the patient has poor balance, the upper part of his body can be dressed while he is lying in bed by turning him from side to side.

If the patient has good balance, the upper part of his body can be dressed while he sits on the side of the bed.

Shoelaces must be tied securely. Elastic shoelaces are best because they do not need tying.

A long-handled shoehorn makes it easier for a patient to put on his shoes.

Food and Fluid

The doctor usually orders a high protein diet to help rebuild the stroke patient's body. In the early acute stage, the patient may be on a liquid diet, with soft solids added as he is able to tolerate them. Later he may receive a regular diet.

At the self-help stage of eating, the patient may need much encouragement because he may be very untidy and clumsy with eating utensils. A damp sponge-rubber mat under a dish will stabilize it. Nonbreakable dishware and drinking cup or glass, a spoon rather than a fork, and a rocker-handled knife may help him to feed himself better. One dish at a time is best at first.

It may be necessary when offering food to a hemiplegic to draw his attention to what is on the plate within the visual field of his affected side. He may be unaware of it and eat only the food he can see. Rotating his plate during the meal brings the food within his range of vision.

Communicating with the Patient

After the onset of a stroke, the patient may be unable to speak and sometimes to understand. It is important to establish a simple way to communicate as soon as possible. This is best done by agreeing to signals and then asking simple questions requiring only "yes" or "no." For example, tell the patient to raise his good hand if his answers to your questions are yes. Phrase questions simply. EXAMPLES: "Are you hungry?" "Are you cold?" "Can you hear me?"

Aphasia

An aphasic is a person with a speech problem. Aphasia is common in a stroke patient. It is important to understand that the aphasic patient has no memory of speech and must relearn speech patterns.

GENERAL RULES

Allow the patient as much freedom to speak as possible.
Let him make mistakes.

Give the patient opportunities to hear speech.

Speak to the patient in short, simple, clear sentences.

Speak slowly.

Encourage the patient to speak and praise his efforts.

Don't force the patient to speak or to see people if he doesn't want to.

Don't talk for the patient.

Don't interrupt while the patient tries to speak.

Don't insist that the patient speak perfectly.

Don't scold if he doesn't speak.

Never become angry. That increases the patient's difficulties.

Don't remind the patient that he could speak before he became ill.

Never isolate the patient.

Don't expect thanks for any attention that you show.

If the patient is doing something, don't interrupt, even though his activity may appear foolish to you.

Don't make unrealistic demands that the patient cannot possibly meet.

Don't allow the patient to be disturbed by unnecessary problems.

Adaptive Equipment

In the course of recovery, a stroke patient may require many pieces of adaptive equipment: a leg brace, special shoes, a wheelchair, an arm sling, and/or a cane.

Infant Care

23

Pregnancy and Hospital Delivery Care

Pregnancy is a normal condition, but the signs of pregnancy may be the same as for some unhealthy conditions. It is therefore important to see a doctor when you suspect that you are pregnant. If you don't have a doctor call your local hospital or health department or county medical society to get the name of a doctor or clinic.

Usual Signs of Pregnancy

a missed menstrual period
tender or enlarged breasts
morning nausea
more frequent urination
more frequent tiring

The First Visit to the Doctor

A medical history is taken.
Blood is withdrawn from a vein for laboratory tests.
A physical examination is done. This includes weight, height, blood pressure, eyes, ears, nose, throat, and teeth.
Heart and lungs are listened to with a stethoscope.
Breasts and abdomen are viewed and pressed.

An internal (pelvic, or vaginal) exam is done.

The doctor explains how to care for yourself during pregnancy, how often he expects you to come in for a checkup, and when to expect the baby.

What to Discuss with the Doctor

> any physical, marital, or financial problem (he can direct you to help)
> any medicine of any kind you are taking (many medicines can affect the embryo)
> weight gain and weight control
> exercise
> sleep and rest
> working
> traveling
> clothing
> bathing
> breast care
> douching
> sex
> smoking
> birth control (past and future)

Lamaze (Method of Prepared Childbirth)

The Lamaze method of prepared childbirth, popular in many parts of the world, is based on the premise that any person can condition his mind to control pain. Both expectant parents attend lectures and films that educate them about the processes of conception and birth. This knowledge calms fears that cause pain-increasing tensions. The expectant mother is taught breathing exercises that help her to consciously release tense muscles during labor contractions. She is taught body exercises that limber pelvic joints, help circulation, and increase elasticity of the pelvic floor. Her husband is taught to help her to control labor pains. Delivery is accomplished with mother awake, baby alert, and father present. For further information read *Painless Childbirth, Thank You Dr. Lamaze*, by Marjorie Karmel, or contact the American Society for Psycho Prophylaxis in Obstetrics, Inc., 1523 L St., N.W., Washington, D.C. 20005.

Planning for the Hospital Delivery

Preparing Home for Your Absence

In the last month before the baby arrives, both parents should take a careful look around the house and decide what special jobs they can do in order to be free of extra chores on the mother's return from the hospital with the new baby. EXAMPLES:

cleaning: closets, drawers, bookcases, stove, and refrigerator
washing: drapes, bedspread, rugs
shopping: for family clothing needs
food shopping and meal planning: for family during the mother's absence and for several days after her return from hospital
cooking: extra food and freezing it for use during the mother's absence and after her return

Collect what is needed for the baby and prepare his area.
Pack a bag for the hospital.
If there are other children and you plan to have an outsider to help while the mother is away, have that person stay with you for a week or so before the mother enters the hospital. Then the family adjusts to her presence and she learns the layout, habits, and routines of the household.

What Is Needed for the Hospital

FOR THE MOTHER
toothbrush
toothpaste
a comb (and brush if desired)
a nail file
hair curlers
face cream
bath powder
cologne
nightclothes (if not furnished by hospital)
slippers
a bathrobe
street clothing

FOR THE BABY
  a shirt
  3 or 4 diapers
  2 or 4 safety pins
  pair waterproof pants
  a sacque set or a kimono or nightie
  socks or booties
  sweater set and cap
  receiving blanket
  outer bunting (if winter)
  a wool blanket

Leaving the Hospital

The hospital nurse and mother will dress the baby.

The nurse will explain the baby's feeding schedule and instruct the mother on preparation for feeding. Most hospitals provide enough formula feedings to last through the first night at home.

The nurse will tell the mother when she is to see the doctor for her own care and when for the baby's care.

Hospital Care of the Newborn

The Delivery Room

After birth the umbilical cord is clamped and cut.

The baby's breathing is started.

The baby's footprints are taken and identification bracelets are placed on both mother and child. This prevents the possibility of mix-ups.

The baby is weighed, measured, and examined.

The baby is bathed and dressed in a clean shirt and diaper.

The baby is wrapped securely and placed head down in a tilted warming crib. This position helps drain mucous from the air passages.

The baby remains in the delivery room as long as the mother is there. When the mother is ready to leave the delivery room, the baby is taken with her if he is "rooming in" or to the nursery.

The Nursery

The baby's temperature is taken each morning.

The infant is bathed each morning with warm oil or soap solution, rinsed with clean warm water, and patted dry with a clean towel or diaper. The baby is dressed in a clean shirt and diaper. A clean sheet is put on the crib. Then the baby is wrapped in a receiving blanket.

Infants are changed before and after every feeding.

The baby's doctor usually examines the infant each morning after its ten o'clock feeding.

Babies are held for all feedings.

Special precautions are taken to care for newborns in hospitals. All hospitals require nursery personnel to have physical exams that include throat cultures, blood tests, and stool examinations.

A baby is usually carried to his mother to be fed. He is changed and swaddled before being taken to her.

If the baby is breast-fed, equipment for breast care is taken along with the infant. The mother's nipple is cleansed just before the baby is put to suck.

If the baby is bottle-fed, the specific formula is taken with the baby. The name on the formula bottle is checked with the baby's name bracelet.

Two clean diapers are also taken. One diaper is placed under the baby's chin during the feeding. The other diaper is placed on the mother's shoulder for use while burping the baby.

The name bracelets of both mother and child are checked before the infant is given to the mother.

The name bracelet of the infant is checked with the name card on the crib before the baby is replaced in the crib.

The color, consistency, and number of times of all urinations and stools are recorded on a daily sheet. This helps the doctor determine the normality and response of the infant to life.

Only a doctor gives information about the baby to the mother or other members of the family.

Only breast-fed babies are taken to their mothers for night feedings. Formula-fed babies are fed in the nursery by the nurse.

Formulas are prepared in a special room apart from the nursery.

Boy babies may be circumcised while in the hospital. Injection of vitamin K, which helps blood to clot, is usually ordered for male infants before circumcision.

All nursery personnel wear caps, masks, and gowns when in the nursery. Other hospital personnel are kept out of the nursery.

Rooming In

Some hospitals have "rooming in," a service in which the infant is kept in the same room as the mother.

A schedule similar to that of the nursery is followed for the baby. The main difference is that the mother takes care of the baby. Hospitals differ as to the amount of care that a mother is expected to give; some hospitals allow full care, including a 2 A.M. formula feeding to be given by the mother. Other hospitals remove the infant during the night.

24

Preparing to Give Infant Care

Infant Needs

Furniture

A full-sized crib with

easily movable casters;
firm, nonsagging springs;
a bed level that requires no stooping;
solid head and foot panels;
closely spaced bars for the sides;
a foot-pedal-release safety lock to raise and lower the sides;
a washable, durable, nontoxic finish;
a firm, waterproof mattress.

A firm crib mattress gives a baby's body proper support so that his bones can grow firm and straight.

The side bars of a crib should be closely spaced so there is no possibility that the infant's head could become wedged in an opening.

A foot-pedal safety lock on a crib is better than a hand release because there is no possibility that the baby can reach the release when he is in the crib.

A nontoxic finish means it contains on poisonous substance.

An infant so quickly outgrows a bassinet that it is unwise and unnecessary to buy one.

A carriage that is

strong and roomy;
nontippable, can be braked safely;
nontoxic;
supplied with safety straps;
easy to handle;
furnished with a firm, wetproof mattress.

It should be large and strong to allow for the growth and increased strength of the baby and to give it maximum protection.

A pillowcase used as the bottom sheet for the carriage mattress stays in place better than a sheet.

A carriage pillow prevents the baby's head from being injured by jars and knocks. The pillow must be secured against the headboard of the carriage to prevent its slipping and covering the baby's face.

A small chest of drawers for the baby's clothing.

A bathinette or firm table on which to bathe and change the baby.

Shelves to hold the baby's supplies.

Clothing

A simple infant layette of soft materials is all that is needed. Clothes should be washable and require little or no ironing. They should have front openings and easy fastenings. Frills, bows, and ruffles should be avoided.

The choice as to whether to use home-laundered diapers, a diaper service, or disposable diapers should be made by the mother in terms of income and baby needs. No one kind of diaper is best. Some mothers use all three: diaper service during times when diaper needs are heavy, disposable diapers for trips, and home-laundered diapers during periods when fewer diapers are needed.

Layette (clothing in size 6 months)
    3 or 4 dozen cloth diapers, if laundered at home
    1 dozen cloth diapers, if diaper service is used, or
    3 or 4 dozen disposable diapers (to be replaced as used)
    6 shirts (cap-sleeved for winter, sleeveless for summer)
    4 nighties
    6 short kimonos or sacques
    2 sweater sets with caps
    2 pairs of socks
    4 pairs booties
    6 receiving blankets

2 full-sized blankets
8 safety pins (for diapers)
2 pairs waterproof pants
1 bunting for winter

Linens and Bath Supplies

FOR THE CRIB
1 full-sized nontoxic bumper
4 fitted bottom sheets
diaper pads (disposable pads are best)

FOR THE CARRIAGE
2 pillowcases for bottom sheets
carriage pillow and case
fasteners to secure pillow
fasteners to secure covering blanket

Do not use a pillow for a mattress or plastic bags as bed protectors. A pillow is too soft to support the baby and it can interfere with the baby's breathing. A plastic bag can suffocate a baby.

FOR THE BATH
2 soft bath towels (large squares are best)
4 soft, thin washcloths (mitts are best)
an apron for you
a tray with:
    a sterile, capped jar filled with sterile cotton balls
    a sterile, capped jar filled with sterile water
    a soap dish
    a bar of mild soap
    another soap dish and soap for diaper pins
    a small jar of alcohol
    a pair of small blunt-edged scissors
    baby lotion or oil
    baby powder
    a soft hairbrush and small comb

Formula Equipment

The choice of whether or not to breast-feed, use formula made at home, or use ready-made formula in disposable bottles must be made by the mother after consultation with her doctor. And it is a choice that cannot always be made before the baby is born. Sometimes a mother who wishes to breast-feed her baby is unable to do so. Or the doctor may change the baby's formula from a ready-made formula to formula made at home. So it is not advisable to purchase full formula equipment before the baby arrives, unless the mother is certain that she will make formula at home. However, she should have three or four bottles with nipples to use for drinking water and orange juice, and except for the measuring pitchers and one of the covered pots, she will need the same equipment as for formula. If she is to breast-feed, she will need some special equipment, perhaps nursing bras, a cleansing tray setup, etc., but these requirements are so individual and doctor's attitudes toward them so different that it is best to wait until after the baby's birth before purchasing any of these things.

Equipment
    12 bottles with caps, tops, and nipples
    a large covered pot with a rack for bottles
    a large covered pot to hold other equipment
    a small covered pot in which to boil nipples
    a pair cooking forceps
    a quart-size measuring pitcher
    a cup-size measuring pitcher
    a set of metal measuring spoons
    an orange juice squeezer
    a metal strainer (small)
    a metal funnel
    a tablespoon
    a table knife
    a bottle brush
    a nipple brush

Miscellaneous Equipment

FOR SOLID FEEDING
    a baby spoon
    a dish
    a cup

FOR DIAPERS
    a covered enamelware or stainless steel diaper pail
    water softener (Borax)

FOR LAUNDRY
a laundry basket
a mild soap powder such as Ivory Flakes
a mild antiseptic such as Diaperene

Arranging and Organizing Equipment

Organize the baby's things to save steps, time, and effort.

Plan the arrangement of the furniture so that it is all together in a unit but no one piece interferes with another.

Plan drawer and shelf space to best suit the furniture arrangements.

Place equipment so that it is in the area where it is most needed. EXAMPLE: Place the diaper pail under the changing area. Store everything for the crib near the crib. Have everything for changing diapers either on or stored near the changing area. Have indoor clothing stored together near the changing area. Store outdoor clothing and carriage necessities together. Store formula equipment together in its own place in the kitchen. Have baby laundry necessities all together. Find an out-of-the way but convenient storage place for the carriage.

Planning Care

The most important things in an infant's life are food and sleep and love.

During the first year of life, a child grows more than at any other time. To support this growth, he needs proper food and frequent feeding. His diet will be ordered by his doctor but you must see that he eats it.

Breast milk or formula is his first food. Then new foods are gradually added, one at a time, and offered in small amounts mixed with formula.

Any feedings should be given in a quiet place when the baby is not overexcited or overtired. You must give the baby what he needs as well as what he likes. Be pleasant but firm about this.

During his first two years, a baby learns nearly three-fourths of everything he needs to know in order to survive. Studies have shown us that the purpose of sleep is to dream, and that through dreaming, a person records learning into memory. If a person gets too little sleep and cannot dream enough, he becomes cross, tired, unhappy, and his resistance to disease is lowered. It is easy to see that an infant who is learning so much so quickly needs proper sleep.

He needs a warm, dry, airy sleeping place that is protected from drafts, bright lights, and loud noises. And he will sleep best if he feels secure. He feels most secure in his own crib and in his own room. He should be put to bed at regular hours and not be allowed to play actively or become excited before bedtime. He should be dressed in comfortable, loose sleeping clothes that do not bind him when he moves.

The other necessity for an infant's healthy development and growth is love. In medicine, this is called TLC, tender loving care. Studies have shown that TLC is so important that no infant can survive without it, and with it the sick and weak can thrive.

Making a Schedule

Consider the baby's natural eating and sleeping patterns. Arrange what needs to be done for him around those patterns. EXAMPLE:

6:00 A.M.	baby wakes up — is hungry
	change diapers and crib linen, if needed
	give formula — burp
	change diapers
	return to crib
	baby sleeps
9:30 A.M.	baby wakes up — is hungry
	give bath
	change clothes
	change crib
	give formula — burp
	change diapers
	return to crib
11:00 A.M.	(while baby sleeps)
	make formula
	do laundry
	ready carriage
2:00 P.M.	baby wakes up — is hungry
	change diapers
	give formula — burp
	change diapers
	dress baby in outdoor clothes
	put in carriage for airing
	take outdoors

5:30 P.M.	baby wakes up — is hungry
	take out of carriage
	remove outside clothes
	change diapers
	give formula — burp
	change diapers
	put in crib
6:30 P.M.	(while baby sleeps)
	remove carriage linen
	put away outside clothes
9:30 P.M.	baby wakes up — is hungry
	change diapers
	give formula
	change diapers
	dress baby for night
	prepare crib for night
	put baby in crib
12:00 midnight	(while baby sleeps)
	change diapers

Safety

Nature protects the fetus, or unborn child. It floats within the mother's uterus or womb in a fluid that cushions it from injury. It is kept at a constant ideal temperature and receives exactly the kind of nourishment it needs. It is secure and isolated from most diseases.

At birth, the infant emerges into a strange, dangerous, indifferent world where its life depends on your thoughtful attention. You must make the infant's new world as safe and satisfactory as his old one was. In order to do this, you must anticipate and avoid dangers. This is not always easy, for danger exists in everything the baby needs.

Older Baby Safety

As soon as a baby starts to use his hands and crawl, he is exposed to new dangers. These must be anticipated and avoided.

Don't leave him alone except in a safe place such as his crib, a playpen, or a fenced-off area of a room.

Use straps to secure him in his high chair, toilet seat, carriage, or in the car.

Allow him in the kitchen and bathroom only when an adult is with and watching him.

Place all medicines, household cleaners, and poisons of any kind out of his sight and reach.

Place matches and cigarette lighters where he cannot get at them.

Place electrical appliances where he cannot turn them off or on, pull them down on himself, burn, or electrocute himself. Put blind plugs in all outlets.

Place sharp objects such as knives or razors out of his reach.

DANGER·	SAFETY MEASURES
	The Crib
Smothering	Never use a pillow for a mattress. Never use a plastic mattress cover. Never use a plastic bag for any reason. Never use a small pillow under the head. Never put pillows or toys in the crib.
Burn	Never use a hot water bottle.
Infection	Wipe the crib and mattress daily with a mild antiseptic. Keep all crib bedding clean and dry.
Poisoning	Use a mattress of nontoxic material.
Malformation	Use a firm mattress. Use a fitted bottom sheet.
Bruising	Use a crib bumper until the baby is old enough to lift it or chew on it.
Falling	Always keep the side rails up when the baby is in the crib.
	The Carriage
Infection	Wipe the carriage daily with a mild antiseptic. Be sure the carriage mattress is firm, wetproof, and of nontoxic material.
Smothering	Use a pillowcase as a bottom sheet. Use a firm carriage pillow behind the head. Fasten it in place so it cannot fall on the baby's face.
Chill	Fasten covers with blanket clips.
Falling	Fasten the safety straps when the baby is in the carriage.

DANGER	SAFETY MEASURES
Running Away	Always place the carriage on a level area, never on a slope.
	Be sure the brake is set when the carriage is at rest.
Tipping	Watch that animals or children do not knock against the carriage.
Collision	Pull the carriage after you when going through a door. Then you can see anything coming.

Clothing SEE: Dressing, Washing.

Infection	Wash his clothes and bedding with special care.
	Give diapers special care; dry the baby's laundry outdoors when possible.
Scratches	Stick diaper pins into a cake of soap when changing his clothing, or fasten them and put them well out of the baby's reach. When fastening his diaper, place the pin crosswise in the direction of the baby's back.
Prickly Heat	Do not overdress.
Chill	Do not underdress.

Bath SEE: Bathing.

Falling	Never leave the baby alone on a table, sink, chair, or other raised place for any reason.
Burn	Never put him near a stove or radiator.
	Be sure the bath water is the proper temperature.
Chill	Be sure the baby is protected from drafts.
Bruising	Never probe in the eyes, ears, nose, or mouth.
Scratches	Never use sharp-edged scissors around a baby.
	Keep his nails clipped short.

Food

Overfeeding	Make a formula and prepare foods exactly as ordered.
Upsets	Always burp the baby after feeding.
Undernourishment, Infection	Keep baby's food equipment separate from other household equipment. Use them only for him.
	Sterilize his formula, bottles, and nipples.
	Wash and scald the tops of milk cans, baby foods, etc., before opening.
	Wash and scald his eating utensils.
	Throw away old or soft nipples and cracked or chipped bottles or bottle caps.
	If breast-fed, be sure mother's nipples are cleaned before nursing.
Cuts	Use unbreakable eating utensils.

DANGER	SAFETY MEASURES
	Anyone Handling an Infant
Infection	Bathe and wear clean clothes daily. Wash hands each time before picking up the baby.
Scratches	Do not wear jewelry, pins, pocket pens or such when handling the baby.
Forgetfulness	Be alert, careful, and accurate in everything you do.
Falling	Always support the infant's head and back.

Place small objects such as buttons, beads, or beans where he cannot find them.

Keep ends of tablecloths and dangling cords out of his reach.

Remove easily broken objects from any area where he is active.

Block open doors and stairways with gates.

Keep him from contact with radiators and hot water faucets.

Keep cribs or beds away from windows.

If windowsills are low, use protective rails.

Toy Safety

Select toys carefully. Any toy can be dangerous if misused. Remember that there is no substitute for adult interest and supervision.

Choose toys to suit a child's age and development. Some toys have age group labels on the package. Heed warnings such as, "Not intended for children under three years of age."

When selecting toys for older children, remember that younger brothers and sisters may have access to them. Avoid giving games and toys that have small points or sharp edges.

Buy stuffed toys and dolls with fabric labels that read "non-flammable," "flame-retardant," or "flame-resistant," as well as ones that read "washable" and "hygienic materials."

Teach the child the proper use of toys. Instructions for use should be easy to read and to understand.

Toys that produce excessive noise such as cap pistols can damage a child's hearing. Avoid them.

Avoid games involving arrows and darts unless the games are supervised by an adult.

TOYS FOR SMALL CHILDREN

Be sure that any toy given to a small child

is too large to swallow;

has no detachable small parts;

cannot easily break into small pieces or pieces with sharp edges;

has no sharp edges or points;

does not have straight pins, sharp wires, or nails that can work out of it;

is not made of glass or brittle plastic;

is labeled "nontoxic" (in general, avoid painted toys for a child who puts things in his mouth);

is not hinged so that fingers can be pinched or hair caught in the toy;

has no long cords or thin plastic bags.

For further information consult the Bureau of Product Safety, 5401 Westbord Ave., Bethesda, Md. 20016.

25

Handling an Infant

Most people feel nervous about handling an infant, he seems so tiny and frail.

Professionals involved in infant care have devised special ways to lift, turn, and hold infants that take into consideration their special needs.

The infant's head always needs protection. His skull is made of sections that have not yet grown together. This open skull is necessary for the birth process, which squeezes and molds the head in its passage through the birth canal. After birth the head bones begin to grow together, but for a long time the baby has two soft spots on the top of his head. The smaller one is on top near the back of the head. This one closes within a month or two after birth. The larger one is on top, near the front of the head, and closes at about eighteen months. Because of these, special care must always be taken in handling the baby's head.

Air bubbles that become trapped in the baby's stomach can be released if the baby is held in an upright position to be burped.

An infant reacts with alarm to only two stimuli. If support is suddenly withdrawn, he will jerk and cry. He will do the same if he hears a loud noise.

Once you learn the special ways to handle an infant, you will never again feel nervous. Always observe the following general rules:

Keep a firm but gentle grasp.
Avoid sudden movements; move the baby smoothly.
Keep the infant's head and neck supported.

Never pull on a hand, arm, or leg.
Keep the baby's nose and mouth uncovered.

Football Hold

Tuck the baby over one of your arms so that his head rests in your outstretched hand, his spine is supported by your forearm, and his buttocks are secured between your elbow and waist.

This is a very good hold for carrying the baby. It leaves one of your hands free to carry something else such as a bottle of formula. This hold is used in most hospitals when a baby is taken to its mother for feedings. It is also used when a baby's head is washed.

Regular Feeding Hold

Sit and hold the baby in your lap nestled in one arm and against your breast. Hold the bottle with your other hand.

To burp, put the bottle aside; use both your hands and lift the baby in the pick-up position to an upright position against your diaper-protected shoulder. Gently rub and pat his back.

Cross-Leg (Mayo) Feeding Hold

Lift your left leg and cross the left ankle over the right knee. Place the baby so that his buttocks are fitted into the hollow between your legs and his feet are against your right waist. This is a very secure position and it frees your left hand. It has the added advantage of lessening the chances of germs passing from you to the baby.

To burp, put the bottle aside and lean the baby forward in a sitting position, supporting his chest, neck, and head against your widespread right hand. Pat his back with your left hand.

Alternate Cross-Leg Feeding Hold

Use a footstool. Keep your right foot on the floor. Place your left foot on the stool so that the foot is in front of your right leg. Position the baby in the same way as for the cross-leg hold. This hold is preferred by those with heavier legs.

Picking Up an Infant

Stand over the infant.

Approaching from one side of the infant, gently insert one of your palms under the back of the baby's head. Spread your fingers

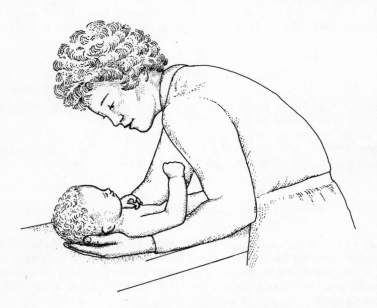

Putting an infant down

so that your hand supports the head, neck, and part of the shoulders.

Approaching from the infant's other side, gently insert your other palm under the infant's hips. Spread your fingers to support the lower back.

Lift the infant in a smooth swing.

Putting Down an Infant

Hold the baby in the pick-up position while lowering him.
Lower the hips until they rest on the mattress.
Remove the hand that supported the hips.
Raise that hand and place it to reinforce your other hand, supporting the baby's head.
Lower the baby's head to the mattress.
Slowly withdraw your hands.

Temperature or Enema Hold for an Infant Under Three Months

Sit in a straight chair. Put a protective pad on your lap. Lay the infant's stomach down on the pad with his head against your thigh. Place your forearm along the infant's spine to restrain him. Use that hand to separate the buttocks. Insert the thermometer or enema tube 1 to 1½ inches with your other hand.

Temperature or Enema Hold for an Infant over Three Months

Sit in a straight chair. Put a protective pad on your lap. Lay the baby, stomach down, across the pad. Reach a hand and forearm under the baby's shoulder to grasp his outside arm. Let his head rest on your forearm. Be sure his nose is free to breathe. Catch the baby's legs between your own. With your other hand, ease the buttocks apart and insert the thermometer or enema tube. Do not insert more than 1 to 1½ inches.

Cradle Hold

The cradle hold is used to transfer the baby from one person to another.

Cradle the baby in your arms so that his head is supported by one of your elbows and his feet by the other.

Have the other person hold his arms in the same position. Hold the baby above the arms of the other person. Settle the baby into his arms, then remove yours.

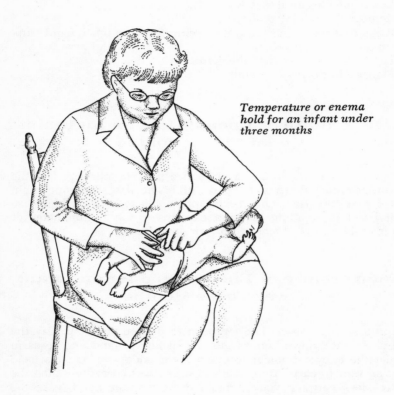

Temperature or enema hold for an infant under three months

Body-Arm Hold for Tub Bathing

Place the baby lying on his back.

Approach him from the same side with both of your hands.

Slip one of your hands under his head and shoulders and grasp his far shoulder and arm in a firm grip. Support his head with that wrist.

Slip your other hand around the lower legs so that they rest in the palm of your hand. Grasp the near leg between your thumb and fingers.

Lift the baby and lower him feet first into the water and a sitting position.

Release your hold on his legs and use that hand to bathe the baby. Keep the shoulder-arm hold until you are ready to wash his back.

When ready, lean the baby forward so that his chin rests on your free arm, then shift the shoulder-arm hold to that hand. Use your released hand to wash his back.

To remove the baby from the tub, use the original hold positions and lift.

This hold is also used when placing a baby on a scale.

Turning an Infant

Method No. 1. Cradle the baby's head in the palm of your hand. Work your same forearm under the baby to support the spine. With your other hand take a gentle hold of the baby's cheeks and chin. Roll the baby over.

Method No. 2. Place one of your hands under the baby's head. Use your other hand to grasp his ankles. Rest his feet in the palm of your hand. Insert your index finger under and between the ankles. Encircle the ankles with your thumb and third finger. Lift slightly and turn the baby toward you. At the same time, slip the hand you are using to support the head forward along the cheek.

Hold for Examining a Child's Head

Two people are needed.

Lay the child on his back with legs extended.

Place your forearm gently across the child's knees (little or no pressure is needed to prevent the child from bending his knees or kicking).

With your other hand take hold of the child's wrists and extend his arms above his head and hold his wrists against the bed. This position braces his head between his arms, so that it is easy for

another person to examine or treat the eyes, nose, mouth or face.
To treat an ear, turn the head before bracing it.

Restraining, or Mummy, Hold

This hold is used if it is necessary to restrain a child under five
years old in order to give him medicine or to examine or treat any
part of his head.

Turning an infant

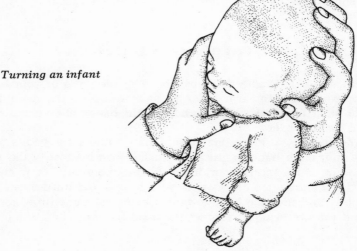

Equipment
    a sheet or blanket sized to the child (it should be long enough
        to extend from the child's shoulders to beyond the feet and
        wide enough to wrap around the child three times)

Lay the sheet in the crib.
Place the child on his back in the center of the sheet so that his
head, neck, and shoulders are above the sheet.
Position the child's forearm lengthwise alongside the body.

Pull the far side of the sheet over the arm to cover the entire body.

Tuck that sheet end securely under the near side of the body, so that the forearm is held in place and the legs are held together and extended.

Position the child's near arm alongside the body.

Pass the near side of the sheet over that arm and around the length of the body.

Continue to wrap it snugly around the body until the sheet ends.

If necessary, pin the sheet end in several places along the length of the body. Be careful to prevent sticking the child.

26

Bathing, Weighing, and Measuring

Bathing

Tub Bath

Equipment
  a plastic apron
  a baby tub or clean kitchen sink
  2 towels and a washcloth
  a padded area on which to lay the baby
  a complete change of baby clothes and a receiving blanket.
  a tray with *a soap dish and mild soap; a baby hairbrush; baby lotion or powder; a jar of sterile cotton balls; a jar of sterile water; a bottle of boiled drinking water and sterile nipple*
  a small bowl or bag for used cotton balls

Be sure the room is warm and draft-free.
Wash your hands and put on a clean plastic apron.
Collect all supplies and take them to the bath area.
Spread one of the towels on a flat surface of the bath area.
Fill the tub a third full with hot water. Test the temperature of the water with a bath thermometer or your elbow. Infant skin is very sensitive to heat and cold and can be burned by water that would not seem too hot to the adult hand. And water that might feel lukewarm to adult fingers could be cool enough to chill the baby. The adult elbow is more sensitive to heat and cold variations than the adult hand. The most acceptable temperature for a baby's bath is 105° F. (40.5° C.).

When everything is ready bring the baby and lay him on the spread towel.

Before undressing him, clean the eyes, nose, and ears with cotton balls over which you have poured sterile water. Use a separate cotton ball for each eye. Wipe only once from the corner near the nose to the outer corner.

Cotton balls and sterile water are used to clean the eyes, nostrils, and ears of the baby because they lessen the possibility of injuring

Body-arm hold for infant tub-bathing

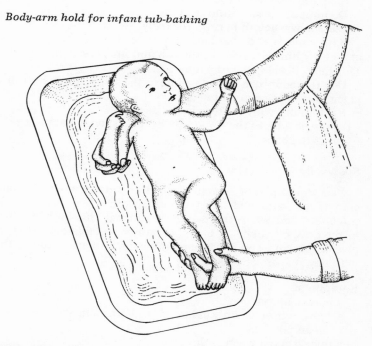

these delicate parts. Q-tips or cotton wrapped on a stick should not be used because, even with very gentle probing, these delicate parts can be injured.

Use a separate cotton ball for each nostril and each ear. Do not probe in the nose or ears.

Make a mitt of the cloth in order to wash the face. Do not use soap on the face. Pat it dry with the clean towel.

Give the baby a few sucks of water from the bottle. Then squeeze his cheeks gently to force the mouth to open.

Look inside the mouth for any white spots. Such spots, which can mean the presence of disease, should be reported to the doctor.

To wash the baby's head, hold him in the football hold with his head over the tub. Use your free hand to soap his head. Rinse it with the washcloth. Pat it dry. Take special care to protect the baby's soft spot (or fontanelle).

Undress the baby.

Use the body-arm hold to introduce the baby into the tub.

Use one hand to hold the baby.

Soap the baby with your other hand.

Do not put the soap into the tub.

Use the washcloth to rinse the baby.

Bath time is exercise and play time. Let the baby kick, squeal, and enjoy himself while in the tub and undressed on the bath area. This helps develop healthy muscles.

Use the body-arm hold to remove the baby from the tub and to place him on the spread towel.

Pat him dry with the towel.

Apply powder in the same way as for a sponge bath.

Dress the baby.

Sponge Bath

You would give a sponge bath to an infant when the umbilical cord is still attached, after circumcision, when the child has an infection, and when the doctor so orders. This bath can be given in the crib, on your lap, or on a counter or tabletop. Wherever you give it, be sure you have enough room to work. Protect the floor with newspapers or plastic.

Equipment
   a plastic apron
   a baby tub or clean kitchen sink, bathroom sink, or a large, clean pot
   2 towels and a washcloth
   a padded area on which to lay the baby
   a complete change of baby clothes and a receiving blanket
   a tray with *a soap dish and mild soap; a baby hairbrush; baby lotion or powder; a jar of sterile cotton balls; a jar of sterile water; a bottle of boiled drinking water and a sterile nipple; a small bowl or bag for used cotton balls*

Be sure the room is warm and draft-free.

Wash your hands and put on a clean plastic apron.

Do not put the soap into the water.

Lay the baby on the table.

Undress the upper part of the baby, keeping his chest and arms covered with a large towel.

Use your hand to soap the baby's arms and chest. Rinse them with the washcloth. Pat them dry.

Apply powder to your own hand and then rub it on the baby. This prevents the baby from inhaling loose powder.

Turn the baby on his side and wash his back in the same manner. Then replace him on his back.

Dress the upper part of the body.

Undress the baby's legs and bottom.

Wash them in the same manner.

GIVING CORD CARE

Cord care is given to the newborn until the umbilical cord falls off and the umbilicus, or navel, heals.

Pour a small amount of alcohol onto a sterile cotton ball and gently dot the umbilical area.

Do not put alcohol on any other part of the baby's body.

Do not put a dressing or bandage over the umbilicus.

CLEANING THE GENITALS OF A GIRL

Pour sterile water over several cotton balls.

Separate the folds of the vulva with one hand.

With the other, hold one of the wetted cotton balls.

Wipe one side of the vulva once from the top toward the rectum in one direction. Discard the ball.

Take a second cotton ball. Wipe the other side of the vulva once from top toward the rectum. Discard the ball.

Take a third cotton ball. Wipe the center of the vulva once from top toward the rectum. Discard that ball.

CLEANING THE GENITALS OF A BOY

Circumcised: Give special care. SEE: Circumcision.

Uncircumcised: Pull the foreskin of the penis back. Use a cotton ball and sterile water to clean under the foreskin.

Apply lotion or powder to the palms of your hands and then gently rub the baby's body.

Finish dressing the baby.

Swaddle him in a clean receiving blanket and return him to his crib.

Sponge Bath for Fever Reducing

For fevers over 104° F. (40° C.)

Equipment
    2 washcloths
    a small basin of ice cubes
    6 diapers or 6 towels
    a bath towel
    a plastic sheet
    a cotton blanket
    a bedsheet
    a washbasin containing tap water (the same temperature as
       the patient's elevated one)
    a pitcher of cold water
    a rectal thermometer for checking patient's temperature
    a bath thermometer for checking water temperature
    boiled drinking water in a baby bottle, cup or glass (lemonade
       may be substituted for older children and adults)
    clean pajamas or other bed clothing

Tell the patient what you are going to do.

Undress the patient and position him flat on his back.

Cover the patient with the cotton blanket.

Place the plastic sheet covered with the bedsheet under the patient so that the bed is protected. SEE: Making a Sick Bed.

Take the patient's temperature.

Make sponge water the same temperature.

Wring out one washcloth from the ice basin and lay it across the patient's forehead.

Soak the six diapers or towels in the basin of tap water.

Wring out four, one at a time, and wrap one at a time around the legs and arms.

Wring out the fifth and turn the patient on his side.

Lay the wet diaper or towel to cover the patient's back and buttocks.

Turn the patient onto his back.

Wring out the sixth and lay it to cover the chest and abdomen.

Change the forehead cloth.

Offer the patient a drink.

Take the patient's temperature.

Add cold water from the pitcher to the basin to lower water

temperature to the same as the patient's current thermometer reading.

Unwrap, soak the diaper or towel, wring it out, rewrap the body part until all have been changed.

Continue repeating the last five steps until the patient's temperature reaches 100° to 102° F. (37° to 39° C.).

Then remove all wrappings and the plastic sheet and sheet cover.

Pat the patient dry with the bath towel.

Put on clean pajamas.

Straighten the bed.

Cover the patient.

Prevent chilling.

Take the patient's temperature after half an hour.

Weighing

It is normal for a newborn to lose weight during the first few days after birth. Because of this, he is weighed daily while in the hospital. This accurate, early weight record enables the doctor to determine how well an infant is adjusting to life and his feedings, and it gives the doctor an opportunity to regulate the feedings to best suit the infant's needs. However, by the time of discharge, daily weighing is no longer necessary.

In fact, most doctors advise against having baby scales at home. They think that the mother who weighs her child too often can become unnecessarily concerned about normal variations in weight. Since an infant is always weighed during any office visit to the doctor, that weight record tells enough to judge a baby's normal progress.

However, there are certain circumstances when a doctor may want an infant weighed at home. Usually he orders that the child be weighed once a week, and that the weighing be done on the same day at the same time.

A scale is always balanced with a diaper or pad in it. This is so that the naked baby is never placed directly on the cold scale, but on the diaper or pad. (The scale must be balanced with the diaper in it so the diaper weight will not be added to the baby's weight.)

A baby is usually weighed naked, so that the weight of clothing is not added to the baby's true weight.

A baby can be weighed with clothing if the clothing is weighed again apart from the baby, and the clothing weight subtracted from the total weight of baby and clothing.

Stand directly in front of the scale when you read it to see the markings straight-on and so read the weight correctly.

Be sure the room is warm and free of drafts.
Wash your hands.
Before weighing, balance the scale with a diaper in it.
Place the naked baby in the scale on the diaper.
Stand directly in front of the scale to read it.
Adjust the pound scale until the balance begins to change.

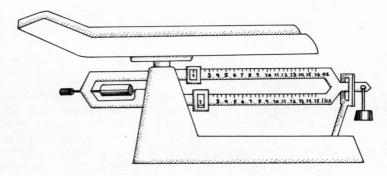

Baby scale. Pounds are read on the bottom line, ounces on the top.

Adjust the ounce scale to balance.
Read the pound scale first, then read the ounces.

1 pound (lb.)	= 16 ounces (oz.)	= 0.4536 kilograms (kg.)
½ lb.	= 8 oz.	= 0.22680 kg.
¼ lb.	= 4 oz.	= 0.11340 kg.
4 of ¼ oz.	= 1 oz.	= 0.02835 kg.

Measuring an Infant's Length

Equipment
   a measuring tape
   Scotch tape
   a straight-edged article, such as a ruler

Use the Scotch tape to attach part of the measuring tape to an even-surfaced tabletop. So there can be no danger of the baby falling, attach the tape near the center and away from the table ends.

Lay the baby on his back alongside the tape so that the top of his head is even with the start of the measure.

Straighten the baby's legs and hold your hand gently across the baby's kneecaps.

Hold the ruler flat against the baby's heels and at right angles across the tape.

Note the tape marking where the ruler crosses the tape.

27

Dressing an Infant

A Closed Garment

Put the garment on feet first. Then lift the baby by his ankles to work the shirt over his buttocks to his chest. Or put the garment on head first, but protect the baby's face with one of your hands by holding your fingers widespread and cupped over the face. Or stretch the garment neck with your hands to frame the baby's face.

Slip your fingers inside one of the sleeves. Find the baby's hand, protect it with your fingers, and draw it through the sleeve. Do the same for the other arm. Be sure to take the baby's entire hand.

An Open Garment

The opening usually goes to the center front. Sometimes there is a side closing.

Slip your fingers inside one of the sleeves. Take hold of the baby's hand and draw it through. Tuck the rest of the garment under his shoulder. Turn the baby on his sleeved side and put on the other sleeve in the same manner. Place him on his back to adjust and fasten the garment.

Do not pin shirts or other garments to the diapers. Pinning restricts the baby's movements and soon tears the garment.

Cuff the bottom of a shirt at the waist of the diaper.

A Blanket

Spread the blanket open in a diamond shape on a flat surface.

Place the baby in the center of the blanket with his head and feet directed toward opposite corners.

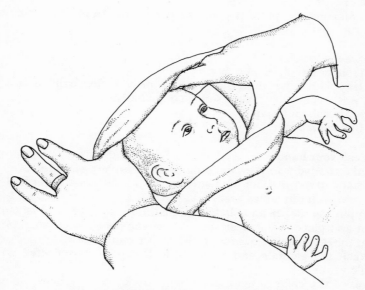

Dressing. Frame an infant's head with your hands when putting on a slipover garment.

Fold the bottom corner up to cover the baby's feet and legs.

Wrap one side corner over his body and arms. Wrap the other corner over the baby.

Let the top corner fall forward to cover the top of his head.

A baby is wrapped in, rather than covered, so that he can't kick off the blanket or pull it over his face to interfere with his breathing.

Changing a Diaper

To fold a diaper, first fold it in thirds and then fold one end to the middle.

A diaper can be adjusted to fit the size of the baby by making the folds larger or smaller.

To diaper girls, place the thicker part under the buttocks (the urine of girls runs to the back).

To diaper boys, place the thicker part to the front (the urine of boys runs to the front).

Equipment
   a table or flat changing area
   a tray with a jar of sterile water, a jar of cotton balls, and a
      waste container for the soiled cotton balls
   a soap dish and soap
   a folded diaper

Wash your hands.

Take the baby to the changing area. It is very easy for even a tiny baby to move about on a surface, so a baby must never be left alone on an unprotected area.

Unpin the diaper and stick the pins into a cake of soap or close them and place them in the tray out of the baby's way. Soap on a point makes the pin go through the diaper more easily.

Wash the genitals and buttocks with cotton balls wetted with sterile water.

Notice the color, amount, and consistency of any bowel movement. These show how well the baby is adjusting to his feedings and to life.

Notice any rash or redness. These can mean diaper rash.

Dry the skin with fresh cotton balls.

Discard all cotton balls in the waste container.

Apply powder or lotion to your own hand, then to the baby.

Place a clean diaper under the baby's buttocks.

Draw the front of the diaper between the legs and up over the genitals.

Adjust the back diaper flap over the front at each side so that the diaper fits snugly.

Pin crosswise, directing the pinhead toward the back.

Don't pin the shirt to the diaper; fold the shirt edge over the diaper.

Take the baby back to his crib. (Never leave the baby alone on the changing area, not even for a second.)

Return to the changing area.

Take care of the soiled diaper and pad.

Clean out the waste container.

Wash your hands.

Report to the doctor any abnormal stool, skin redness, or rash.

Infant Urine Specimen

Equipment
   a plastic sandwich bag
   nonallergic (hypo-allergenic) skin adhesive tape

Open and fanfold the sides of the sandwich bag to form an oblong cup.

Position the cup lengthwise over the genital area and under the hips.

Secure the cup in place by taping it to the skin.

A good time to apply such a specimen collector is just before a feeding. An infant will usually void during or just after a feeding. Also the act of holding the infant for feeding maintains the baby in a semi-erect body position, which allows urine to drain into the container.

Washing Baby Clothes

A baby's clothing requires special care in order to protect his delicate skin from rashes, burns, and germs. These general rules should be followed.

Wash baby clothes apart from other household laundry.

Do not use bleach, enzymes, or strong detergents. They are irritating to the baby's skin.

Give extra rinses.

Clothing and Bedding

Baby sheets, towels, receiving blankets, shirts, and all cotton clothing may be washed together, but apart from other household laundry, in an automatic washer. Use a mild soap such as Ivory Flakes. Rinse three times and dry thoroughly in an automatic dryer or in fresh air and sunshine.

Woolens, such as sweaters and blankets, must be washed by hand in a cool solution of mild soapsuds. Rinse three times in cool water. Wrap in a towel and gently knead. Then spread flat on a dry towel, stretch to the right shape, and let dry in the shade. Putting woolens into hot water makes them shrink and mat.

Waterproof pants, if not machine washable, should be washed by hand and aired frequently.

Soiled Diapers

Keep a covered enamelware diaper pail near the place where you change the baby.

Keep the pail half filled with water and Borax (see package label for correct amount; Borax is a water softener that helps remove urine and bowel movement from diapers).

Clean the diaper pail and change the Borax solution at every diaper washing time.

Place wet diapers in the pail as soon as removed.

Rinse soiled diapers by holding them in the toilet bowl while flushing the toilet. Then place them in the diaper pail.

If using a washing machine, you need not launder diapers every day; every other day is often enough. Daily washing wastes time, water, and soap.

Wash the diapers with a mild soap or detergent.

Rinse at least three times. A mild antiseptic, such as Diaparene, may be added in the last rinse. This rinsing prevents diaper burn.

Dry thoroughly in an automatic dryer or outside. Putting a damp diaper on an infant can chill him.

Fold without ironing.

Diaper pads and some brands of waterproof pants may be washed with the diapers.

Diapers should be boiled occasionally. When this is done, wring diapers from the hot, soapy wash water and place them in the cleaned diaper pail containing a mild soap solution. Bring to a boil and boil ten minutes. Rinse diapers four times and dry in the sun and air if possible. Boiling sterilizes diapers. It kills the germs that resist usual laundry methods. Boiling also whitens diapers.

28

Feeding an Infant

Nutrition

Before birth a fetus stores minerals such as calcium and iron for use immediately after birth. Breast milk or formula are therefore sufficient for the newborn, providing adequate calories, food value, and fluid.

Within the first few months, the baby's doctor may order cereal and orange juice.

Later the doctor will suggest introducing egg yolk, strained meats, strained cooked vegetables, and strained cooked fruits to suit individual needs.

Use of canned or bottled strained and chopped baby and junior foods is sometimes advised against by modern doctors. Studies have shown that many of these foods have added salt and sugar that can be harmful to a baby's health. As a result of these studies, some brands of baby foods have discontinued adding those substances to their products. If in doubt, read the label or consult your doctor. Vegetables, fruits, or meats prepared at home are certainly fresher and better for a person of any age. Electric blenders make the food preparation for infants an easy process at home. Vegetables and fruits should be soft-cooked in a covered pot in as little water as possible and without salt, sugar, or spices. The cooked vegetable or fruit is pureed in the blender and is then ready for the infant to eat. Meat, chicken, or fish should be trimmed of all bones and fat and soft-cooked in a covered pot in as little water as possible. No salt, sugar, or spices should be added. The meat, chicken, or fish and the liquid in which it cooked should be pureed in the electric blender before offering it to the infant. If no blender is available, foods prepared in the same way can be mashed through a strainer.

When the child outgrows the need for strained food, food can be chopped in the blender or mashed with a fork.

A new food should be introduced at a time when the baby's appetite is keenest. If the baby rejects a new food, do not force it. Wait several days and offer it again.

Finger foods should be offered as soon as a child shows a desire to feed himself.

Caloric Requirements

A toddler needs 45 calories for each pound of body weight a day.
A two-year-old requires from 1,000 to 1,500 calories a day.
A preschool child requires from 1,400 to 1,800 calories each day.
A schoolchild requires 1,500 to 2,500 calories each day.

SAMPLE MENU FOR A ONE-YEAR-OLD CHILD

6 A.M.	Juice (fresh orange is best)
8 A.M.	(Breakfast) Cream of Wheat or Cream of Rice with milk
10 A.M.	Milk
12 noon	Soft-boiled egg
	Chopped spinach
	Mashed potatoes
	Gelatin or mashed fruit such as banana
	Milk
3 P.M.	Milk
	Cheese cubes
5:30 P.M.	Canned junior foods or fresh vegetables and chicken, lamb, or liver that has been chopped in an electric blender
	Applesauce
	Milk
7 P.M.	Milk

Water should be offered often during the day at other than mealtimes.

Breast-Feeding

Breast-feeding is an easy and natural way to feed a baby. Besides providing complete food and protection from infection and allergy, breast milk is easily and rapidly digested. Breast-feeding also establishes a special closeness with the newborn that gives emotional satisfaction to both mother and child. A breast-fed baby is more content and healthier. He sleeps better, gains weight faster, and has fewer gastric upsets and less constipation than a formula-fed infant. Breast-feeding may require some effort at first but it is usually very successful. Even women with adopted children have been able to produce breast milk and breast-feed.

Before the true milk comes in, the nursing baby gets colostrum, a yellowish fluid that is rich in immunity factors. This milk comes in between the second and the sixth day after birth. As the colostrum disappears, the milk looks less rich, but it is the baby's perfect food, with all the nutrients and protective factors in exactly the right proportions.

Breast-fed babies prefer a two- to three-hour interval from the beginning of one feeding to the beginning of the next. This is more frequent than formula feeding but has good results, for the more you nurse, the more milk you produce. Nurse the baby on one side for about ten minutes, then switch to the other side for as long as the baby wants to suck. At the next feeding offer the baby the last-used breast first and switch to the other. Don't rush the feeding. The infant's need to suck is as great as his need for food.

Nipple Care

Nipple care should start several months before birth and continue for the first few weeks of nursing. Massaging salad oil or hydrous lanolin into the nipple and the surrounding area for five minutes daily will help prevent dry, cracked, and bleeding nipples. Pulling gently on the nipples during this time will bring them out so the baby can get a good sucking hold. Exposure to air and sunlight helps toughen the nipples. Wearing a well-fitted nursing bra provides support and comfort to the breasts. Plastic bra liners can irritate the nipples. It's better to pad the nipples with clean handkerchiefs if leaking is a problem.

Washing the nipples once a day with clean water is sufficient to clean them. Avoid using soaps, alcohol, or other types of cleaners. They can dry and irritate nipples.

Holding for Breast-Feeding

Hold the baby in any position that is comfortable for both of you. You may want to lie down for some feedings and sit for others. Night feedings can be given in your bed with a minimum of disturbance to all. There is no danger if you or your husband fall asleep. The baby will love it.

Offering the Breast

Support the breast with one hand and press it back from the nipple with your thumb and forefinger. This makes the nipple easier to grasp and also keeps the breast away from the baby's nose so that he can breathe easily. Draw the baby close until his cheek touches your breast and the nipple is next to his mouth. He will turn his head toward it and open his mouth to find it. Then pull him closer, so he can get the entire nipple in his mouth and suck.

To remove the baby's mouth from the nipple, gently press the breast away from the corner of his mouth until the suction is broken.

Give a gentle burping pat on the back when you switch breasts or when the baby is finished nursing. If he falls asleep, don't burp him but lay him down on his side or stomach.

Most healthy, full-term, breast-fed babies do not need solids for four to six months. Giving them too early could mean a decreasing milk supply and a greater risk of allergy.

Sometimes, however, a doctor may decide that nursing is inadvisable. In conditions such as heart or kidney disease, tuberculosis, or a mental or nervous disturbance, breast feeding would be a strain on the mother. Even if a women were healthy, a doctor might decide against breast feeding if she had less than half the milk the baby needed, if her nipples cracked and bled, or if the baby were born weak or deformed.

A doctor may order a formula as well as breast feeding.

He might order a complementary formula if the mother did not have enough milk to satisfy the baby.

He might order a temporary formula if nursing were interrupted for a day or two.

He might order a substitute formula to be used if the mother had to be away for one or more feedings each day.

Mother's Diet for Breast-Feeding

A nursing mother requires more protein and more calories than usual. Her diet is very important. She must be very careful to eat the right foods so that she can offer the infant the food substances he needs for healthy growth.

She needs a quart of milk a day. If she tends to gain weight, she may use part of the quart of milk in cooking and substitute skim milk for whole milk.

She needs large servings of fish, poultry, meat, eggs, or cheese at least three times a day.

She needs one large glass of orange or grapefruit juice (preferably fresh) and another helping of fresh or canned fruits each day.

She needs one large fresh salad and one helping each of a green and a yellow vegetable each day.

She needs small quantities of butter or margarine and salad oil.

After these foods have been planned into her menu, she can and should have such carbohydrates as cereals, breads, and potatoes.

If she feels hungry or weak, she may need between-meal snacks. Fruit or milk make good snacks.

She should avoid spices and use stimulating drinks such as alcohol or coffee in moderation. Sweets and rich foods should be very limited. A nursing mother should never take medicine or laxatives without the knowledge and approval of her doctor.

Spices, coffee, alcohol, medicines, and laxatives can pass into the milk and affect the nursing baby.

Other Care for Nursing Mother

A mother should get plenty of rest and be free from emotional upsets. Too many visitors, long visits, or other exhausting activities should be avoided. An afternoon nap while the baby sleeps is helpful. Daily exercise in fresh air eases tensions and the mother will eat and sleep better.

The doctor should be told if the mother develops sore or bleeding nipples. He may take the baby off breast feeding.

The doctor should be told if the mother develops engorged or caked breasts. He may advise using a breast pump or expressing milk by hand.

Expressing Milk by Hand

Cup the breast in your hand.

Place your thumb above and your forefinger below the nipple on the edge of the dark skin area around the nipples.

Squeeze thumb and finger together. *Don't* slide the finger and thumb out toward the nipple.

Change the positions of your fingers several times so that you reach all the milk ducts that radiate from the nipple.

Alternate breasts every few minutes.

Don't worry if no milk comes at once; with a little experiment and practice you will be able to express it.

La Leche League

This is an international organization of mothers who dispense information about breast feeding and give encouragement to other mothers who are breast feeding. There are local chapters throughout the United States. For further information call your local chapter (listed in the telephone book) or write to La Leche League International, 1916 Minneapolis Ave., Franklin Park, Ill. 60131.

Demand Feeding

Many doctors today think that each baby should set his own feeding schedule. These doctors order feedings "on demand," which means that the baby is fed any time he cries or makes sucking mouth movements — his signs of being hungry.

However, if the baby cries, it does not always mean that he is hungry. You should search for other causes for his crying before feeding him.

Change his diaper.

Look for open safety pins.

Check his skin for chill or overheating.

Burp him.

Change his position.

Pick him up and cuddle him.

Then, if the baby still acts hungry, feed him.

The baby may demand an early feeding: if he vomited the last feeding, if he did not finish the last feeding, or if the feeding was not rich enough or of sufficient quantity.

Sucking and Thumb Sucking

Doctors once thought that thumb sucking could affect mouth and tooth formation and was not good for the baby. They also discouraged the use of pacifiers, but these attitudes have changed.

A few years ago, Scandinavian doctors developed a camera that takes photographs of a fetus within the uterus. Some of these pictures show unborn babies sucking their thumbs and indicate that thumb sucking is natural and necessary. Today most doctors allow thumb sucking and pacifiers, and suggest a long feeding time for the baby to satisfy his sucking needs.

Whatever the method of feeding, whether breast or bottle, allow enough uninterrupted time to let the baby eat and suck to contentment. He should have thirty minutes for feeding and sucking at each feeding.

Preparing for a First Feeding

Equipment
    formula or sterile water
    a clean bowl
    clean measuring spoons
    a clean knife for measuring

Measure 1 tablespoon of formula and put it into the bowl.

Measure 1 teaspoon of dry baby cereal and add it to the formula in the bowl.

Mix well until slightly thickened.

Adding the cereal to the formula makes a smoother mixture than adding formula to cereal.

Formula Feeding

Many babies are fed on a formula ordered by the doctor instead of being breast-fed. Formula is a substitute for mother's milk and a doctor tries to make the substitute as much like mother's milk as possible.

Unless the baby is allergic to them, the doctor orders a formula made from three ingredients: milk, sugar, and water. He has a wide range of milk products and sugars from which to choose.

He considers the general condition of the infant and decides on a particular milk and a particular sugar, in amounts that are best for the individual baby.

Even so, he may need to change the infant's formula several times before he finds one on which the baby thrives.

It is most important that you notice how the infant reacts to his formula and report to the doctor any of the following signs that suggest the formula may not be agreeable.

The baby does not take all the feeding. (Sometimes he may leave a small amount, but if he leaves the bottle unfinished at every feeding something is wrong.)

He cries more than usual or acts as though he has abdominal pain.

He finishes a feeding too quickly or acts hungry soon after finishing one.

His bowel movements are loose and frequent.

His bowel movements are constipated and infrequent.

He spits up or vomits more than normally after feeding.

The doctor gives a written order for the baby's formula. It tells the exact measurements for each ingredient, the amount to be given at each feeding, and how often the baby should be fed. The doctor will usually order 1½ to 2 ounces of formula for each pound of the baby's weight.

Whether the baby is fed on breast milk or formula, the doctor always tells the mother how often he should be fed.

Underweight infants or premature infants are sometimes fed every two hours.

Most newborns are fed every four hours through the day and night, that is, at 6:00 A.M., 10:00 A.M., 2:00 P.M., 6:00 P.M., 10:00 P.M., and 2:00 A.M.

By the time the normal infant leaves the hospital or shortly afterward, the doctor orders the 2:00 A.M. feeding discontinued.

The 10:00 P.M. feeding is the next to be discontinued by the doctor.

A formula order looks like this:

12 oz. H_2O
4 oz. EM
1 T. DM #3
$4 \times 4 \times 4$

This means 4 ounces to be given in 4 feedings at 4-hour intervals, that is, 6:00 A.M., 10:00 A.M., 2:00 P.M., and 6:00 P.M.

oz. = ounce.
H_2O = water.
EM = evaporated milk.
DM #3 = Dextri-Maltose #3. Dextri-Maltose is a simple sugar often used in formulas. It is canned in three varieties: No. 1, plain Dextri-Maltose; No. 2, ascorbic acid is added to the Dextri-Maltose; No. 3 soda bicarbonate is added to the Dextri-Maltose.

Other milks that may be ordered for formula:
condensed milk
whole milk
powdered milk
skim milk

Other sugars that may be ordered for formula:
granulated or table sugar
corn syrup, such as Karo
brown sugar

Water used in formula should always be sterile.
There are many commercial powdered milks made only for babies. Some of them are

Alacta;
Lactum;
Olac;
Olactum;
Similac.

Giving a Formula Feeding

If formula is ordered others may sometimes feed the baby, but the mother or father should give the feeding as often as possible.

Feeding, sucking, and holding are part of the necessary tender, loving care that make a baby feel secure and well. The baby's satisfaction from the fulfillments of TLC are related to the person who gives it. The mother and father should have the major share of that delightful relationship.

Wash your hands.

Take the filled bottle from the refrigerator.

Place the bottle upright with a cap unscrewed in a pan of hot water in a bottle warmer. Keep the water well below the cap. The warming water should never be boiling. It is quite warm enough at 120° F. (50° C.).

Get two clean napkins or diapers to use as a bib and as protection while burping the baby.

After ten minutes remove the bottle from the hot water.

Keep the bottle upright while putting a sterile nipple in the feeding position.

Test the temperature of the formula by shaking a few drops onto the inner wrist. It is the correct temperature if the drops cannot be felt as either hot or cold.

Formula should never be tested by holding the bottle against the inner wrist. This tells you only how warm the bottle is, not the warmth of the formula.

Place the pan of hot water and the formula near the feeding chair.

Wrap the baby in a receiving blanket and take him to his changing table.

Change his diaper.

Rewrap the receiving blanket.

Pick up the baby and sit in a comfortable chair. Hold the baby in a semi-upright position that is comfortable for both of you.

Put one napkin under the baby's chin, the other over your shoulder.

Upturn the bottle into feeding position.

See that the neck of the bottle is filled with fluid so that no air gets into the nipple. Air can be swallowed. It causes gas pains or colic and can make the baby take less feeding or spit up a good part of it.

Touch the nipple to the baby's mouth. He should immediately root his mouth to it.

Allow a half an hour for feeding. See that this time belongs only to the baby.

You can adjust the rate of flow on a regular baby bottle by tightening or loosening the twist of the cap. Judge the rate of flow by the bubbles. The speed at which bubbles rise into the bottle of formula as a baby sucks shows how quickly the baby is taking the feeding. Bubbles should not rise too rapidly; if they do, the cap should be tightened or the hole might be too big and the nipple should be changed.

Burp the baby when he has finished half the bottle. Hold him upright against your shoulder, that is protected by the diaper. Gently massage his back. Allow five minutes for burping.

If the baby falls asleep during feeding, wake him with gentle flicks of your finger against the soles of his feet. Gently push and pull the nipple into and out of his mouth. Burp him again.

The bottle can be replaced in the warm water during the burping period. Retest the formula temperature before feeding.

Burp the baby again at the end of the feeding period.

Change his diaper if necessary.

Put the baby back in his crib. Place him on his side or stomach so that any formula he might spit up can drain freely from his mouth.

Rinse out the formula bottle and nipple. Milk is a good breeding place for germs; rinsing prevents germ growth.

Put all equipment away.

Some doctors advise against warming formula bottles before feeding. These doctors think such warming increases the growth of undesirable bacteria in milk. Follow whatever method the baby's doctor orders. Unwarmed formula is usually removed from the refrigerator and allowed to stand at room temperature for twenty minutes before feeding.

Preparing Baby Formula

All formula is sterilized by boiling to prevent the possibility of infection.

There are two methods of boiling formula: Method 1, when the formula is prepared under clean conditions, put into the bottles, and then the bottles are boiled; and Method 2, when everything used in making the formula is boiled before the formula is prepared.

Method 1 is the easiest and the one most often used. However, all formulas cannot be made by this method as some milk products curdle if boiled for long periods. Method 2 is used to prepare formulas made from such milk products.

A twenty-four-hour supply of formula is made up at one time.

Three extra bottles, two for drinking water and one for orange juice, should be prepared at the same time as the formula.

Be sure to measure all ingredients exactly.

To measure liquid, set the measuring container on a flat surface and stoop to see the fluid at eye level.

Boil extra nipples for emergency use. Store them in a sterile, covered jar. An extra nipple may be needed if a nipple on a bottle proves unsatisfactory or becomes unsterile.

Boil the nipple jar and cover, and other jars, such as those for sterile water and cotton balls, along with the formula preparation.

Keep all equipment used in making formula together and apart from those for other household use.

Scrub an unopened can of milk with soapy water and scald it with boiling water before opening.

If canned liquid milk is used, open a fresh can to make each batch of formula. Any leftover milk can be used in cooking for other family members.

Take care when using canned powdered milk to have the can open only when measuring for each batch of formula. Clean the connecting area between the top and the can daily. Use a cotton ball and alcohol to clean it.

METHOD I (USUAL METHOD)
Equipment
 a teakettle or large pan for boiling the water for the formula
 a large pot with a lid
 tongs
 a bottle brush
 a nipple brush
 a measuring cup
 measuring spoons
 a pitcher or a quart-size jar
 a towel
 a table knife
 a can opener
 long-handled spoons
 a small jar with a cover (for extra nipples)
 a small covered pot for nipples and caps

Follow the same rules for scrubbing the bottles, nipples, and other equipment.

Set your clean equipment up on the counter.

Measure the needed amount of water directly from the faucet.

Add sugar or syrup and stir well until dissolved.

Measure and add milk.

Stir well until dissolved.

Divide the formula into the right number of feeding bottles.

Set the nipples, caps, and tops on the bottles. *Do not screw tops on* because the buildup of heat during the boiling period can cause the bottles to explode.

Set the bottles upright in a large pot.

Prepare two bottles of water, taking it from the faucet.

Prepare an empty bottle for orange juice, if needed.

Set these bottles in the pot also. (Remember not to screw caps on.)

Put a nipple jar and cover and the tongs in the pot.

Put two inches of water in the pot.

Cover and bring to a boil.

Time for twenty minutes after boil starts.

Remove from stove.

When the bottles are cool enough to touch, remove them from the pot.

Screw the caps on tightly.

Let cool before refrigerating.

Prepare extra nipples by placing them in boiling water in the small pot for three minutes.

Use tongs to remove them to the sterile jar at the end of the boiling time.

METHOD 2 (USED ONLY WITH CERTAIN MILK PRODUCTS)
Equipment

    a teakettle or a large pan for boiling the water for the formula

    2 pots with lids, large enough to hold all the bottles

    tongs

    a bottle brush

    a nipple brush

    a measuring cup

    metal measuring spoons

    a pitcher or a quart-size jar

    a towel

    a table knife

    a can opener

    a long-handled spoon

    a small jar with a cover (for extra nipples)

    a small covered pot for nipples and caps

Wash your hands.

Put on a clean apron.

Put water on to boil in the teakettle.

Put water on to boil in the small pot.

Scrub the bottles and nipples with brushes in hot soapy water. Nipples should always be tested during washing and those with too-large holes should be thrown out.

Rinse them thoroughly.

Allow the bottles to drain dry. Don't wipe.

When the water in the small pot is boiling, add the nipples and caps. Boil three minutes only. Longer boiling makes the rubber soft and crack.

When nipples have boiled three minutes, take them off the stove and drain at once. Set the pot aside with the cover on.

Put all other equipment into the two large pots. Put the bottles in upside down so the water will rise into them. Put the tongs in last so that you can remove them easily.

Add two inches of water.

Cover and put on to boil. After the boiling point is reached, time the boiling for five minutes.

When the teakettle and large pots have boiled for five minutes each, remove them from the stove and allow them to cool with their covers on. When cool enough to handle, take off the pot lids and lay them upside down on the counter. Do not touch the insides of the lids.

Remove the tongs with your hand. Then use the tongs to remove the other equipment.

Place the bottles and pitcher and measuring cup upright on the counter.

Use the sterile tongs to remove and place the other equipment in the sterile, inverted pot lids.

Lay the prongs of the tongs in the inverted lid. Be careful not to contaminate them. Rest the unsterile handles on the tabletop outside the lid.

Mix the formula in the large pitcher.

First put in the ordered amount of water.

Use the measuring spoons to add the sugar or syrup. Stir with the long-handled spoon until fully dissolved. Sugar is always added to water so that you can watch it dissolve. Undissolved sugar can cause uneven distribution of sugar among the feedings, so that one can be an overrich formula feeding and another underrich.

Add milk last.

Stir until completely dissolved.

Divide the formula into the bottles. You can be sure you have measured the ingredients accurately if the whole amount divides into equal and ordered amounts in each bottle. Don't touch lips of containers together when pouring liquids.

Make two bottles of boiled water.

If you are interrupted during the making of formula and do not remember whether or not you measured or added any ingredient of the formula, throw that batch of formula out and measure the ingredients again. Otherwise you may make a formula that is too rich or not rich enough for the baby.

Use the tongs to remove the nipples from the small pot and place them on the bottles.

Use the tongs to remove and place the discs and bottle caps.

Screw the tops on loosely.

Put the bottles in cold water for ten minutes.

Screw the tops on tightly.

Refrigerate until needed.

Clean the equipment and put it away.

Disposable bottles

A disposable bottle, such as the Playtex Nurser, is sometimes used in preference to a standard glass baby bottle.

The Playtex Nurser has a bottle-shaped plastic frame designed to hold a disposable presterilized plastic bag.

The bag is attached to the frame with the help of an expander. The neck of the bag is fitted over the expander and then the expander is inserted into the frame so that it clamps the bag in place.

Special nipples that closely resemble the human nipple are used. As the baby sucks the nipples and drains the milk, the plastic bag collapses, lessening the chance of air getting into the baby's mouth.

CARE OF THE PLAYTEX NURSER

Scrub all parts of the Playtex Nurser in hot, soapy water using a bottle and nipple brush. Rinse thoroughly and scald.

Nipples, caps, and expander may be sterilized by putting them into boiling water for three minutes.

Sterile Playtex bottle bags should be kept in their closed box in a clean, dry storage place.

Wash your hands well before placing a bag on the expander.

Fit the neck of the bag well up on the expander.

Be careful never to touch the inside of the bag.

Insert the closed bag end into the holder, then clamp the expander down onto the holder rim to fasten the bag.

Hold the formula or milk to be poured into the bag well above the rim. Do not touch the rim of the nurser with the bottle or pitcher from which you pour.

Touch only the outer edge of the nipple when placing it on the nurser. Put the cap on over the nipple for storage.

When you remove the cap, put it on the bottom of the nurser.

Commercially Prepared Formulas

Today, there are several brands of ready-made formulas on the market. These are sterile and come in disposable bottles. They can be obtained from a drugstore on a doctor's order. They are becoming increasingly popular for both home and hospital use.

29

Growth and Care

Growth is a complex process involving the physical, mental, emotional, and social development of an individual. If any basic needs are not met, underdevelopment occurs.

Growth is a continuous process, occurring from conception to old age, and whatever affects it at one stage will affect all future stages. Learning ability is often dependent on age development.

Growth is an individual process. No two children even within the same family develop at exactly the same rate. Certain general conditions, however, are known to affect many individuals. Height usually increases in the spring; weight usually increases in the fall. An individual's position within a family affects his growth rate. The family "baby" is often that for all of his life.

The usual learning process involves one skill at a time. A child may temporarily abandon one skill in order to learn another. However, once something is learned, it is easily recalled. Learning also requires sufficient freedom to investigate new interests and possible skills. Overprotection can produce a spoiled, weak-willed, or anxious child.

Normal Development of the Newborn

Weight

During pregnancy, the doctor attending the mother checks on her weight and regulates her diet and exercise so that the baby, at birth, weighs about seven pounds. Then the infant is small enough to deliver easily but developed enough for healthy survival.

The normal newborn loses weight during the first few days of life but regains it by the seventh to tenth day.

Height

The average length of a newborn is from 18 to 22 inches.

As a general rule, large parents have large babies and small parents have small babies, but this is not always so.

Appearance

The head seems large for the body and is about a fourth of the body length. The head is the heaviest part of the body. It is sometimes swollen and elongated after delivery but it soon returns to a normal shape. This is because the skull bones have not yet grown together.

The separation of the skull bones can be felt as two soft spots on the top back and front of the infant's head. These soft spots are called the fontanelles. The back one closes first at about a month and a half after the baby's birth; the front fontanelle closes when the infant is about eighteen months.

The newborn's head can be bald or he may have hair of any color or amount, curly or straight. Newborn hair gradually falls out and is replaced by new hair that may differ in color and texture.

The eyes are slate blue but change color at six weeks to six months. The eye muscles are weak and the eyes often cross and uncross. For a few days after birth a newborn's eyes may be puffy and reddened from the eyedrops administered in the delivery room.

The ears are usually small and set close to the head.

The nose is small and soft. Mucus is present and sneezing occurs.

The mouth and sucking instincts are well developed. The chin recedes.

The neck is short, creased, and weak. Shoulders are small and sloping.

The back is curved and limp.

Hands are well formed and can grasp or spread. Nails are paper-thin and sharp.

Legs are froglike and active. Feet are flat and still developing.

The chest and abdomen are round. Sometimes the breasts of either sex are swollen, but this condition soon goes away.

The tied umbilical cord stays until the seventh to the tenth day.

It gradually dries and falls off. This cord is the connecting tube between the baby and the placenta. During pregnancy, the placenta is attached to the wall of the uterus. It is "born" after the baby and is often called the afterbirth.

The genitals of both sexes appear overlarge.

The skin is loose, peeling, and reddened even in the dark-skinned infant. At birth, a layer of substance that looks like cold cream covers the body. This substance has helped protect the fetal skin from the fluid inside the uterus. It also eases the fetus's passage through the birth canal. The fluid is often called the "bag of waters."

Sensory Development

Sight: Reacts to bright lights and large objects.

Hearing: Jerks after loud noises.

Smell: Is thought to be present at birth and to help the baby find his mother's breast.

Taste: Is not highly developed.

Touch: Will grasp anything placed in his hand. The lips are very sensitive. The baby will cry if he feels he is not held securely.

A newborn loses weight in the first few days of life because it is not yet adjusted to being outside the mother's uterus or to taking nourishment by mouth. The intestines of a newborn are filled with a black, soft, tarlike substance called meconium. The meconium must be eliminated from the baby's body by bowel movements before the baby can receive nourishment from his feedings. For the first twenty-four hours after birth, instead of milk, a mother's breasts secrete a fluid (colostrum) that stimulates bowel movements in the baby.

Behavior

The baby reacts to pain and fear. He is born with two fears, loud noises and falling.

If restrained, he will try to free himself. He will try to swim if put into water. But all of his activities, whether sleeping, eating, crying, coughing, or sneezing, are instinctive. He does not remember and is too young to be taught.

Like all animals, he has an individual sense of timing that will form his habit patterns. He begins to show it soon after birth.

His language is crying. He cries when hungry, afraid, under tension, angry, in pain, or in need of affection. The cries are so much alike it is often difficult to learn the cause of his crying, but all of his cries mean something. No baby under three months cries without cause. No baby under three months can be spoiled. Don't be afraid to hold, rock, or soothe him.

Care of the Newborn to Three Months

The baby should be held for all feedings. Propping should be done only in an emergency. If it is ever necessary, place the baby on his stomach in the crib with his head turned to one side and the bottle secured next to his head. If done in this stomach position there is less danger of the baby's inhaling spit-up milk.

No feeding should be rushed. Allow thirty minutes for feeding and sucking.

If the infant falls asleep during feeding, tap gently on the soles of his feet.

Formula must be exactly prepared and sterilized. Reaction to the formula should be noted.

After every feeding, position the baby in his crib on his side for about a half hour. Support his back with a rolled receiving blanket. An older infant who is able to lift his head can be placed on his stomach.

Wrap the infant snugly, but not so tightly as to restrain him.

Keep people with infections or emotional upsets away from the baby; he can react with diarrhea and vomiting. If a baby is tense he frets, squirms, makes sucking motions, holds himself stiff, moves about in the bed, cries, etc.

Sucking relieves his tension. A pacifier soothes him.

Sudden temperature changes can cause skin discoloration and shivers. You can tell whether a baby is at the right temperature if his skin is warm and pink but not sweating. Keep him at a regulated temperature and dress him for temperature changes.

Keep his clothing dry and loose to protect his sensitive skin. Take care in washing his clothing so as to prevent rashes and burns.

Offer him additional drinking water when immunization shots begin (usually after one month). This helps reduce the baby's reaction to the serum.

Prepare a schedule based on the baby's normal sleeping and eating patterns and follow it as closely as possible. He responds best to routine.

A Sample Routine for a Baby on Four Feedings

6:00 A.M.	change wet clothing
	feed and burp (receives milk only)
	change diaper
	place baby on his side in his crib (alternate sides)
	nap
8:30 A.M.	change diaper
9:00 A.M.	orange juice and vitamins if ordered; burp
	mouth care
	bath
	playtime
	change crib
10:00 A.M.	change diaper
	feed and burp (include cereal and fruit if ordered)
	change diaper
	nap
10:30 A.M.	(while baby naps)
	make formula
	do baby's laundry
	ready supplies
	do any chores
2:00 P.M.	change diaper
	feed and burp (include strained vegetable and fruit if ordered)
	change diaper
	playtime
	nap: If weather permits take the baby outside for his nap. If the weather is poor, dress the baby in warm clothes and open the nursery window.
6:00 P.M.	playtime
	change diaper
	feed and burp (include strained foods if ordered)
	change diaper
	put to bed for the night

Change diaper twice during the night without waking the baby.

Normal Development at Three Months

The baby urinates about eighteen times a day.

He has two to four bowel movements. If breast-fed, these are light yellow, pasty, mushy, and sour-smelling. If he is on cow's-milk formula, they are yellow, puttylike and do not cling to the diapers.

He has learned to
   roll from side to side but not roll over;
   stare at his hands;
   play with his hands;
   hold his rattle;
   push his feet against a person's lap or the floor;
   make different cries for pain, hunger, and anger;
   coo and make soft sounds;
   stay awake for longer periods, but he still sleeps most of the time;
   raise his head for longer periods in both prone and supine positions;
   smile when spoken to.

Weight

The baby should double his birth weight in six months.

Height

He should grow four to eight inches.

Appearance

He holds his head upright and moves it from side to side in a full swing of the neck.

He progresses from being propped in a sitting position for ten to fifteen minutes to being able to sit without propping for thirty minutes or longer.

He is interested in people and things around him.

He holds a toy and examines it with his eyes and mouth.

He transfers an object from one hand to another.

He reaches out to grasp what he sees.

He has a decreasing desire to suck and becomes willing to drink from a cup.

He enjoys his daily routine.

Sensory Development

He sees colors and his eyes follow movements.

He looks when someone enters the room and spends much time in looking.

Habits

He sleeps through the night without waking for a feeding, but still has three daily naps: early A.M., late A.M., and early P.M.

Additional foods in his diet change the color and consistency of his stools. One to two bowel movements daily are normal.

He may change gradually from formula to whole milk.

Emotional Development

He has a happy disposition, laughs, recognizes members of the family, and needs company.

He progresses from not minding being with strangers in strange places to resenting being left alone and fearing strangers.

Care of the Four-to-Six-Month-Old Baby

General Care

See that the baby spends most of his waking time among people.

Put him outdoors, if possible, for one of his naps.

String toys across his crib so that he can practice looking and grasping.

Increase the length of his bath so that he has ample playtime.

If necessary, his bath hour can be changed to fit his sleep and the household patterns.

Place him on his stomach often. He enjoys this position and it can keep him from rubbing a bald spot on the back of his head.

Care for teething problems as they develop. They can cause loss of appetite, restlessness, change in feeding habits, and objection to any change in routine.

Do not start toilet training yet. He is still too young.

New foods should be introduced as the doctor orders, and one at a time. Then if a reaction occurs, the doctor will know which food has caused it.

As immunizations continue, don't add new foods to his diet for several days after each injection. In this way, a doctor can quickly determine the cause of any reaction.

Feeding

Jarred foods: Warm by placing the jar in a pan of hot water and letting it stand for ten minutes. Stir. Serve fruit at room temperature. It is not necessary to warm food, but warming gets the baby adjusted to hot foods.

Bananas: Mash with a fork until smooth. Add a few drops of warmed formula to soften.

Egg yolk: Hard-cook an egg for twenty minutes. Then mash the yolk with a fork and add a few drops of formula.

Normal Development from Seven to Twelve Months

The baby progresses from sitting alone for short periods to pulling himself to a sitting position, to creeping, then crawling, then standing.

At about nine months he learns to pull himself to a standing position, but cannot sit himself down.

He likes any kind of self-movement.

He progresses from attempting to pick things up, then holding them with widespread fingers, then to banging things up and down. When he has learned to use his thumb and index finger to pick up objects, he likes to feed himself in this way. He also tries to help dress himself.

Later he pokes and pushes. Still later, he learns to wave bye-bye, and to take things from a container.

Last, he learns to release what he can hold. When he does, he enjoys throwing everything onto the floor.

He develops signs of memory and may cry, laugh, or imitate on demand.

At ten months he can tell the feelings of those who take care of him from the tone of their voice.

He becomes more and more independent and can obey simple commands.

Sensory Development

By nine months, he sees into the third dimension. At one year, his eyes coordinate and he shows pleasure or displeasure at what he sees.

Habits

At seven months, he needs only two naps a day, and by twelve months has shortened or stopped the morning nap. As his ability to move develops, he becomes so involved in all of his new discoveries that he will not want to go to bed.

Emotional Development

The seven-month-old is frightened by separation from his mother.

Care of the Seven-to-Twelve-Month-Old Baby

General Care

Place the baby in a safe, spacious area, such as a playpen, where he can develop his movement abilities.

Select new clothing for the baby that will protect him when he is crawling and also from drafts. Stretch overalls are best.

As soon as he begins to stand, he should have well-fitted shoes.

Allow him to stand and walk only on a firm surface so that his feet develop normally.

Let him practice using his voice, grasping, and watching.

Let him enjoy a variety of interesting toys. These should be large, light, washable, and unbreakable, with a nontoxic finish. Good toys are blocks, soft dolls, hard rubber objects, balls, pie tins, and measuring spoons.

He will put everything in his mouth, so keep all small objects out of reach.

Let him spend plenty of time with people. Play music for him and teach him simple games like patty-cake.

Take him for rides in his carriage to a variety of places.

Teething may be a problem.

Put him to bed at naptime and bedtime whether or not he seems ready or wants to go.

Bathe him in the family tub and change his bathing time to evening.

Bowel training can be started when he shows physical readiness.

Eating

Sit him in a high chair for meals.

Give him unbreakable and washable eating equipment. A dish with a rim helps prevent spilling.

Give him a large bib.

Give him finger foods (such as zwiebach) and his own spoon. Offer diced foods or peas and carrots on his tray. He wants to feed himself and will enjoy trying.

Bring him to the family table at mealtime and give him a portion of the family meal, such as egg or mashed potatoes.

Bowel and Bladder Training

Attitudes toward bowel and bladder training vary. Some doctors suggest that bowel training be started when the baby has a movement at the same time each day, usually after a meal.

Other pediatricians advise against any training until the child shows, by mental and physical signs, that he is ready to be trained. Between the ages of one and one-half and two, the child becomes aware of his ability to move his bowels. At about the same age he may begin to stay dry for two-hour intervals. Then, all doctors agree, he can be trained.

Train him to use either a potty chair or a special seat that fits over the family toilet seat. The chair is more comfortable but the toilet seat accustoms him to the toilet.

Leave him in position for ten to twenty minutes.

Don't flush the toilet while he is on it. It may frighten him and make him resist training. Don't give suppositories or enemas to stimulate a movement.

Praise him if he has a movement.

Never scold if he doesn't have one or if he soils his diaper or training pants.

30

Care in Unusual Conditions

The Premature Infant

Forty weeks is about the normal length of human pregnancy. But pregnancy sometimes ends before this time. When it does end early, special terms are used, depending on the age of the embryo or fetus.

Abortion. The ending of a pregnancy before the first three months and before the embryo or fetus is developed enough to live. The ending may occur from natural causes or may be deliberately induced.

Miscarriage. The ending of a pregnancy after the first three months but before the fetus is developed enough to live.

Premature delivery. The ending of a pregnancy in the later months when the fetus is developed enough to live and does live.

The causes of premature delivery are numerous and not always understood. However, there are certain common conditions that cause labor to start before full term.

Some of these conditions are: illness of the mother during pregnancy, improper placement of the placenta, multiple births, any serious threat to the baby's life inside the uterus, or early rupture of the bag of waters.

The illness of a mother during pregnancy can cause very serious problems. Some illnesses may activate premature labor. Others, such as German measles, may cause changes in the development of the fetus so that the child is born with birth defects.

The uterus is like an inverted pear-shaped balloon. If the placenta, or afterbirth, attaches itself to the uterus across the opening of the cervix or uterine neck, bleeding and premature labor will occur when the uterus enlarges.

Although it can stretch to a very large size, the uterus can hold only a limited weight. Too much pressure on the neck of the uterus forces it to open.

When there is more than one fetus in the uterus, the pressure on the neck of the uterus is much greater.

The premature baby, sometimes called a premie, is very frail and weak. He may weigh between 1½ and 5½ pounds. He is much shorter than the normal infant and his general structure is smaller. Small veins show through the delicate skin and there is no spare fat on his body. The body is often covered with fine, silky hair. The abdomen appears swollen. Fingernails and toenails are soft and short. He may have no eyebrows or eyelashes. Sometimes the skin appears yellow.

The premature infant is put into an incubator immediately after birth. The incubator is especially designed to meet his specific needs. The temperature inside can be finely regulated. A controlled oxygen mixture can be piped into it. The infant is isolated from the possibility of infection. The incubator can be brightly lit for better observation.

Everything is done for the infant within the incubator. He is bathed, examined, medicated, and fed there.

He needs more frequent feedings, sometimes every two hours around the clock. His sucking instinct may not be well developed and he may be fed by a gastric tube introduced through the nose into his stomach. A mixture of water and sugar is usually his first food. When the baby has had a chance to adjust to life outside the uterus, an easily digested milk is added.

The premature infant sleeps most of the time. Any attention he requires is given quickly and only the necessary done, so that his sleeping time will be sufficient. He must be watched constantly. His lungs and crying instinct are not very developed and cannot be relied upon to warn of dangerous changes in his condition.

The baby is allowed to go home when he reaches about 5½ pounds and the doctor is satisfied with his condition. Home conditions should be safe and healthy to receive him.

His care continues to require much time.

He will still need more frequent feedings and may take longer to feed.

He will have more frequent stools.

Regular infant clothing may seem too large. Shirt sleeves and diapers may be folded or cut to fit, whichever the mother prefers.

He should be dressed more warmly than the full-term baby. Temperature changes should be avoided.

He should be kept away from sick people and crowded places.

He will continue to need more sleep and rest.

He will need more frequent checkup visits to the doctor.

He will be slower in physical growth.

He will not sit, stand, or walk as quickly as the full-term infant.

His mental growth will be slower but eventually equal to that of the normal child.

His emotional development is not affected.

He needs TLC as much as any child.

Twins

If a schedule is important for one baby, it is even more important when there are two. Planning your work is essential, for while it is not true that twins are twice as much trouble as a single baby, they do necessitate more work.

So organize your work with care. A mother needs as much rest as she can get. And you will have to train other family members, for they will have to help you.

Feeding is usually the major problem, because twins are often smaller than average and need more frequent feedings. If there is a family member who can help with all the feedings, then the twins can be fed at the same time. Otherwise, one twin should be fed on a schedule that is an hour earlier than the other. Each should be held for all feedings and only in emergencies should bottles be propped.

Formula feedings are usually easier for the mother, but she may want to nurse. In that case, the doctor usually orders a substitute formula. Each baby is nursed at alternate feedings and the one not being nursed receives a bottle feeding.

Often, one twin is stronger than the other. Then the doctor may want the mother to nurse only the weaker. Or if both are on formula, one may require richer formula and more frequent feeding than the other.

In such cases, although the same equipment may be used and the formulas prepared at the same time, care must be taken not to confuse the bottles at feeding time. When one formula is prepared, the side of each bottle should be marked with the name of the twin for whom it is intended and those bottles kept together in the refrigerator but apart from the other twin's bottles.

Care must also be taken not to confuse the twins. They should wear some identification, such as a name bracelet, and each crib should be marked with its owner's name. The use of different colors in the clothing of each is also helpful, particularly if one wears the same color consistently.

Clothing may be washed together. Diapers may be washed together and, if done at home, should be laundered daily. Diaper service is very helpful and so are disposable diapers. Both are expensive with twins.

Baths can be given one following the other. One bath tray setup is all that is needed, but the tub should be scrubbed between babies and fresh water, clean towels, and a clean washcloth used for each. The mother and other family members should think of the babies as individuals and not as "the twins." They should not always be together or do the same things. The family should avoid dressing them alike or comparing one to the other in conversation. See that each fits into the family life as other brothers and sisters do.

The Sick Child

Any changes in a child's normal behavior can mean the onset of illness. If the baby seems cross, fussy, irritable, drowsy, refuses to eat, cries, keeps turning his head, pulls at his ear, draws up his legs, is disinterested in play, vomits, or has diarrhea, he may be sick. You should follow these general rules as soon as a baby shows any combination of the above-mentioned signs.

Take the child's temperature and write it down, together with his symptoms, before reporting to the doctor. It is not abnormal for an infant to run a sudden high temperature. This is because an infant has not developed resistance to many diseases.

Keep the child as quiet as you can. You may need to rock or hold him until he sleeps.

Keep other family members away from the child until he is examined by the doctor. Follow the doctor's orders about further precautions.

If the child vomits or has diarrhea, give him only cooled, boiled water by mouth until the doctor orders otherwise.

Do not give any medicine or treatment unless it is ordered by the doctor.

Medicine may be mixed with fruit or food but never with formula. Mixing medicine with milk could turn the child against milk.

Keep a time-and-description record of temperatures, bowel movements, urinations, vomiting, sleep, and the food and fluids taken.

Calm the child's and family's fears about the illness.

A child who is recovering from illness needs interesting but quiet things to do. Toys and games and records that suit his age are good. He should have each, one at a time. Songs or stories read or told are always enjoyed. He should have nothing that overtires him. Television or radio should be limited to programs that will not overexcite him.

Food should be offered as his appetite demands and every effort made to fix his trays with foods he likes, served in attractive ways. The child should never be forced to eat, and food should be offered in very small amounts.

Long or chronic illnesses can cause a child to lose spirit. Unless treated carefully, he may learn to enjoy his illness. Overanxious parents may make the child anxious. Spoiling may make him demanding.

Preparing a Child for a Hospital Stay

A child should be told that he is going to the hospital and what will happen to him there. He should be allowed to ask questions; these should be answered in simple, matter-of-fact terms that prepare him without fear for what will happen. Several children's books are presently on the market that tell stories about entering hospitals so that a child can identify himself with that situation. The child's doctor or the hospital may suggest a specific book or way of telling the child. Such a presentation of information arouses the child's curiosity rather than his fears.

In addition to telling him, doctor and nurse play kits with make-believe thermometers, needles and syringes, blood pressure cuffs, and other examination and treatment objects allow a child to express curiosity and interest through a doll or another person.

Most hospitals today allow the mother or other relative to stay with and take care of a child during the time that he is hospitalized. This certainly relieves strain on both the child and the parent and allows the parent to learn any special nursing procedures that the child may continue to need once he has returned home.

Most hospitals allow a child to bring a favorite toy to the hospital.

He will feel very possessive of his belongings during his hospital stay.

Many hospitals have playrooms for children to use during their stay. There is usually a skilled supervisor who chooses the kinds of toys and materials that allow a child to express himself regardless of handicaps. Being with other children also lessens the child's conception that he is being singled out for illness.

When a child is confined to bed, a hospital often provides a play companion who brings suitable arts and crafts, puzzles, games, and hobby work such as stamps to the bedside. The companion, who may be a therapist or volunteer worker, helps the child select only activities at which he can succeed and not overtire himself.

Play is extremely important for a sick child. It can distract his pain, fill time between hospital routine and visiting times, and help him to adjust to his illness and express his feelings about it. Playtime can develop new skills and interests and stimulate continued growth.

Schooling is also provided for children requiring unusually long hospitalization or special training to compensate for handicaps.

Television is provided, usually on a limited time basis only, and only for such programs as suit each child's special needs and interests.

Common Unhealthy Conditions

Allergy

Cause: Unknown. Emotional problems play a part.

Signs: Sensitive reactions to agents in food, animals, materials, dusts, pollens, medicine, and a variety of other things that show as asthma, hay fever, eczema, or other skin rashes.

Care: The doctor does a study of the patient and his family history to determine the cause of the allergy. Emotional factors are researched and an effort is made to change them. The agent causing the allergy is avoided, if possible. If impossible, the patient is given injections to help him build up a tolerance to the agent. He is also given antihistamine medicine to control symptoms.

Birthmarks (Nevi)

Cause: Unknown.

Signs: Moles, strawberry marks, or skin discolorations.

Care: Some of these disappear without treatment. Some are removed by doctors. Watch any birthmark for signs of growth and report such growth to the doctor.

Colic

Cause: Gas or an undeveloped digestive system, tension in the family, excitement, noise.

Signs: Hard abdomen, knees drawn up, piercing cries, tight fists.

Care: Offer warm boiled water to drink. Burp the baby. Massage the stomach in a gentle fashion. Comfort, rock, soothe, and pet the baby. Follow the doctor's orders about giving a warm enema or hot water bottle.

Constipation

Cause: Improper food or too little fluid.

Signs: Hard stools.

Care: Increase the fluid intake. Offer more fruit, vegetable and oil; if no results, give a mild laxative or an enema.

Cradle Cap

Cause: Lack of proper head care.

Signs: Dirty yellowish crusts on the scalp.

Care: Keep the head clean. Wash it daily to prevent cradle cap from forming. Apply lotion or oil to loosen crusts. Comb the hair with a fine-tooth comb.

Croup

Cause: Upper respiratory infection.

Signs: Hoarseness, barking cough, difficult breathing (usually occurs at night or early morning), rapid pulse, slight cyanosis (blueness) of lips and fingernails.

Care: Give warm moist air by croup tent, croup kettle, or steamy bathroom. If the bathroom is used, warm the bedroom before returning the patient to it and put dry clothes on the patient.

Dehydration

Cause: Not enough fluids in the body. May result from high fever, diarrhea, vomiting, aspirin poisoning.

Signs: Hot, dry skin; rapid, deep breathing; concentrated weight loss; sunken eyes; pallor.

Care: Follow the doctor's orders.

Diaper Rash

Cause: Urine too acid or too alkaline, bacteria acting on ammonia in the urine, improper washing or rinsing of diapers, use of strong detergents and bleaches in washing diapers, diapers not changed often enough, allergy.

Signs: Redness and sores or pimples on skin in diaper area.

Care: Prevent by proper diaper care. Expose skin to air and light. Change diapers promptly. Boil diapers or rinse with a mild antiseptic such as Diaperene. Use a salve if ordered by the doctor.

Diarrhea

Cause: Infection in the intestine.

Signs: Frequent, liquid, yellow or green stools; pallor; rapid pulse; dehydration.

Care: Follow the doctor's orders. He may order medication or a diet change or both.

Eye Congestion

Cause: Medicine dropped in eyes at birth, infection.

Signs: Puffy lids, bloodshot eyes, discharge from eyes.

Care: Follow the doctor's orders.

Food-Rash Eczema

Cause: Allergic reaction to a food.

Signs: Red, itchy rash. If severe, the skin is thick, scaly, oozing, and crusted.

Care: Follow the doctor's orders. Introduce new foods one at a time. Keep the baby from scratching. Prevent infection of the rash.

Handicaps

Such as defect of a limb, harelip, cleft palate, some heart conditions, deafness, blindness, muteness, mental retardation, cerebral palsy, muscular dystrophy, emotional disturbance.

Cause: Birth malformation, illness of the mother during pregnancy, disease, accidents.

Care: The patient should be encouraged to do as much as possible for himself.

Community agencies can help — for instance, social workers, the welfare department, a public health nurse, the library, specific disease funds.

The doctor may order special treatment by a physical therapist for exercise therapy, a hydrotherapist for water therapy, a recreational therapist, or an educational therapist.

Psychological treatment is very important and should aim at giving the person a sense of security. He should be treated as naturally as possible and as a sharing member of his family.

He should be given as much love, understanding, and patience as he needs, but he should never be pitied. He should be watched for signs of depression, fear, anxiety, suicidal tendencies, or over-gaiety (euphoria) that indicate emotional or mental distress.

Hernia

Cause: Weakness of the muscle wall. May occur in the groin, umbilicus, or diaphragm.

Signs: Swelling or lumps on the abdomen over any of the named areas.

Care: Report to doctor and follow his orders.

Hiccups

Cause: Spasms of the diaphragm (large muscle in the chest cavity).

Signs: Interrupted breathing.

Care: Offer boiled water to drink. Change the child's position. Burp him. If the spasms persist, report to the doctor.

Mental Retardation

Cause: Birth malformation, illness of the mother before birth, disease, accident, genetic oddities.

Care: Special training is necessary to help the child develop the best of his ability. He must be protected from any danger to himself or others. He must be protected from any danger from others. He needs the same love and attention as a normal child.

Noisy Breathing (Snoring)

Cause: Mucus in nose or throat. This is very common in babies. It is usually not serious and is outgrown.

Care: Turn the baby on his side or stomach to drain the nose.

Prickly Heat

Cause: Hot, humid climate, overheating or overdressing, perspiration irritation.

Signs: Small red pimples usually appear in the folds of the body or where clothes fit closely to the body.

Care: Prevent spread by bathing the body often and dressing the child in cool, loose clothing. Expose the skin to air. Keep the skin dry and powdered. A cornstarch bath is soothing.

Rheumatic Fever

Cause: Streptococcus infection.

Signs: Loss of appetite, loss of weight or failure to gain weight, rapid pulse, pains in joints and muscles. Can cause high fever, swollen and painful joints, muscle stiffness in the hands and feet.

Care: Follow the doctor's orders. Keep the child happy and occupied.

DANGER! Rheumatic fever sometimes causes a serious heart involvement called rheumatic heart disease.

Ringworm

Cause: Fungus infection under the skin.

Signs: Small, reddened, scaly patches about the size of a nickel appear on any part of the body, but most often in the scalp and on the legs and arms.

Care: Follow the doctor's orders. Maintain cleanliness to prevent spread.

Swollen Breasts (Newborn of both sexes)

Cause: Glandular changes in the mother just before birth.

Signs: Enlarged breasts, milk droplets.

Care: It disappears of its own accord within a few days. Don't squeeze!

Swollen Scrotum (Newborn male)

Cause: Glandular changes.
Sign: Enlarged scrotum.
Care: It disappears of its own accord within a few days.

Teething Problems

Cause: Irritation of the gums caused by a growing tooth.
Signs: Drooling, fretting, desire to chew on hard objects.
Care: Give a hard rubber or frozen teething ring for chewing. Hard baby teething–biscuits also help. Replace old nipples with new hard ones. Give additional water. See that the baby makes up any loss in sleep or diet that may occur as a result of being off schedule from teething fretfulness.

Tongue-tie

Cause: Cord that holds the tongue is too short.
Signs: Difficulty in sucking, inability to stick the tongue out of the mouth.
Care: Usually given in hospital after birth. The doctor snips the cord with a pair of sterile scissors. Watch for signs of inflammation (it seldom occurs).

Tonsillitis

Cause: Chronic infection by a streptococcus or staphylococcus germ.
Signs: Repeated attacks of sore throat with swollen tonsils, difficulty in breathing, snoring.
Care: Follow the doctor's orders. Sometimes he treats the attacks with antibiotics; sometimes he removes the tonsils and adenoids.

Vaginal Bleeding (Newborn female)

Cause: Glandular changes in the mother just before birth.
Sign: Small show of blood from the vagina.
Care: It disappears of its own accord within a few days.

Worms (Intestinal pinworms)

Cause: Infection through unclean toilet habits or from materials such as towels or underwear.

Signs: Anal itching, white worms visible in stools.

Care: Follow the doctor's orders. Use precautions to prevent spreading. See that the child washes his hands often. Boil his underpants.

Appendices

A

Health Care Glossary

abduction	movement of a part of the body away from an imaginary midline.
abortion	an early end to a pregnancy.
abrasion	a rubbing away or scraping of the skin.
abscess	a localized collection of pus in a cavity.
acute	sudden and severe.
adaptive equipment	devices such as a hearing aid or long-handled tongs that allow a patient to regain use of a body part or to perform a body function.
adduction	movement of a part of the body toward an imaginary midline.
allergic reaction	an abnormal reaction to a substance, such as pollens, certain foods, and medications.
ambulatory	not bedridden; able to walk.
anemia	reduction in the number of red cells, of the hemoglobin content, or of both, in the blood.
anterior	front.
antidote	a remedy for poisoning.
anus	the outlet for the rectum.
aphasia	loss of the ability to speak.
arthritis	a painful inflammation of joints.
atrophy	a wasting or lessening of ability.
axilla	armpit.
bacteria	microscopic organisms.
bladder	a hollow organ in which urine collects.
bland diet	soft, without spice and roughage.

buttocks	fleshy areas of the lower part of the back that cover the hip joints.
cardiac	pertaining to the heart.
cataract	a condition of the eye that impairs vision.
catheterize	to introduce a sterile tube into the bladder to withdraw urine.
Cheyne-Stokes	a type of respiration that often precedes death.
chronic	of long duration.
circulatory system	the movement of the blood through the heart, veins, arteries, and capillaries.
colostomy	an operation by which the large intestine is made to open onto the abdomen.
coma	a state of unconsciousness.
compound fracture	a broken bone protruding through the skin.
condom	a rubber sheath worn on the penis.
contaminated	in the presence of germs.
contusion	a bruise.
convulsion	involuntary spasms or contractions of big muscles.
cyanosis	a blueness of the skin due to a lack of oxygen.
cystitis	an inflammation of the urinary bladder.
cystoscope	an instrument used to examine the interior of the urinary system.
debilitated	extremely weakened.
decubitus ulcer	a pressure sore or ulcer.
defecation	the discharge of feces. Also called bowel movement.
dehydration	a condition resulting from severe loss of fluids from the body.
depression	a state of morbid unhappiness.
dermatitis	an inflammation of the skin.
diabetes	a disease caused by the inability of the body to produce enough insulin, a glandular secretion.
diagnosis	the determination of the patient's condition or the cause of an illness.
diarrhea	frequent loose or watery stools.
digital stimulation	finger massage of the anus to induce a bowel movement.
dislocation	the displacement of a bone.
disoriented	in a confused state of mind.
dysentery	a severe diarrhea.
edema	the accumulation of fluid in the tissues.

elimination	the process of getting rid of body wastes.
emaciation	a wasted, lean, body condition.
emesis	vomiting.
epilepsy	a nervous disease marked by recurring convulsions and loss of consciousness.
evaluation	the determination of physical, mental, and emotional health.
excrete	discharge waste matter.
extension	straightening a part of the body.
feces	the excretion of the bowels. Also called stool.
femur	a bone extending from the hip to the knee.
fetus	an unborn child after the first three months of a pregnancy.
flatus	intestinal gas.
flexion	bending a part of the body.
fontanelle	a soft spot in the skull of an infant.
gastric	pertaining to the stomach.
genitalia	the external sex organs of the male or female.
geriatrics	the study and care of elderly persons.
gynecology	the study of female reproduction, sex organs, and their diseases.
hematoma	a darkened area of the skin containing blood.
hemiplegia	paralysis of one side of the body.
hemorrhage	the escape of blood from a blood vessel.
hemorrhoid	piles; varicose veins of the anus or rectum.
hernia	a weakness in a muscle wall that allows an inner body part to break through it.
hydrotherapy	treatment by water.
hypertension	high blood pressure.
immunization	the process of making a person less susceptible to a disease.
incontinence	the inability to control the elimination of feces or urine.
infection	the invasion of body tissues by disease organisms.
inflammation	a condition characterized by redness, pain, heat, and swelling.
inhalation	the drawing of air or other vapors into the lungs.
isolation	the separation of one person (or object) from others.
Medicaid	a program in which federal, state, and sometimes local governments share the costs of certain medical services.

Medicare	a federal program in which certain health insurance benefits are given to people who are sixty-five or older.
mental health	the state of being able to function under ordinary daily pressures without feeling great fears, confusion, or nervousness.
obesity	fatness.
orthesis	braces or other devices placed on the body for the treatment of a physical disability.
pallor	paleness.
paralysis	the loss of the ability to move, or to feel sensation in, a body part.
passive exercise	the movement of a person's body by a force outside of himself (another person or a machine).
penis	the male sex organ.
physiotherapy	diagnosis and treatment with heat, massage, and manipulation.
posterior	back.
projectile vomiting	sudden forceful vomiting.
prone	lying face down.
prostatectomy	removal of the prostate gland in the male.
prosthesis	an artificial replacement for a missing part of the body.
rectum	the last eight to ten inches of the large intestine.
regurgitation	the spitting up of undigested food.
rehabilitation	methods used to restore the use of body parts after loss.
remotivation	renewal of interest in living.
resocialization	a renewal of interest in being with other people.
restraint	a binder to prevent self-injury.
scrotum	the genital sac of the male.
sedative	a medication that calms an excited patient.
self-care	the ability to dress, groom, and feed oneself.
senile	pertaining to old age.
shock	an upset caused by inadequate blood circulation resulting in lowered blood pressure; a rapid, weak pulse; and pale, clammy skin.
stool	feces; a bowel movement.
supine	lying face up.
testicles (testes)	the two male reproductive glands located in the scrotum.
therapeutic	relating to the treatment of disease.

transfer	move from one location to another.
umbilicus	the navel, or belly button.
ureter	one of two tubes leading from the kidneys to the urinary bladder.
urethra	the tube leading from the urinary bladder to the surface of the body.
uterus	the female organ in which the embryo develops.
Velcro fastener	a self-sticking type of clothes fastener.
voiding	urinating.
vulva	the external female sex organs.

B

Measurements

The following table for liquids is approximate. One liter is not the exact equivalent of one quart, but is 1.056 quarts, and a pint of all liquids does not weigh exactly a pound. It is sufficiently accurate, however, for all but the most precise measurements.

cc.	cubic centimeter	oz.	ounce
ft. or ′	foot	pt.	pint
in. or ″	inch	qt.	quart
l.	liter	t	teaspoon
lb.	pound	T	tablespoon
ml.	milliliter	yd.	yard

$$1 \text{ ml.} = 1 \text{ cc.}$$
$$30 \text{ ml.} = 30 \text{ cc.}$$
$$250 \text{ ml.} = 240 \text{ cc.} = 8 \text{ oz.} = 1 \text{ measuring cup}$$
$$500 \text{ ml.} = 480 \text{ cc.} = 16 \text{ oz.} = 1 \text{ pt.}$$
$$1000 \text{ ml. (or } 1 \text{ l.} = 950 \text{ cc.} = 32 \text{ oz.} = 1 \text{ qt.}$$
$$3 \text{ t.} = 1 \text{ T.}$$
$$1 \text{ pt.} = 1 \text{ lb.}$$

$$12 \text{ in.} = 1 \text{ ft.} = 30.48 \text{ centimeters (cm.)}$$
$$18 \text{ in.} = 1\frac{1}{2} \text{ ft.} = 45.72 \text{ cm.}$$
$$36 \text{ in.} = 3 \text{ ft.} = 1 \text{ yd.} = 91.44 \text{ cm.}$$

C

Patients' Rights

Until recent years an adult patient was expected to be passive and childlike in accepting health care conditions. If a person consulted a doctor or health service, he was not always treated with consideration, not always told what was wrong, or not advised fully about treatment. Today such attitudes are thought to be infringements of civil rights. Being a patient should not deprive a person of basic freedoms. Now the adult patient is thought of as a consumer rather than as a recipient of health services. The rights of a health consumer are

the right to a full disclosure of all facts contributing to the diagnosis and treatment of one's condition, including the possible side effects of medicines.

the right to know what is going on, to question any point, to demand explanation, and to consent to or refuse any treatment.

the right to refuse the services of any one doctor or other health worker and to request a different person to treat or help him.

the right to confirm or challenge one doctor's diagnosis or recommended treatment by seeing another doctor who may be unknown to the first. (Today many doctors suggest such a course of action. Some labor unions will not pay medical claims without such confirmations.)

the right to personal privacy and confidentiality. Discussions about the patient, his condition, or life status should take place only where they cannot be overheard by other than the patient and authorized personnel.

the right to be treated with dignity and respect. No adult patient should be addressed as a number, by his first name, by a nickname, or in any discourteous way.

the right to refuse to participate in a research program; when consenting, the right to full information about the purposes, uses, and methods of the research.

the right to refuse any visit to one's home. When possible, such a visit should be by appointment and at a time convenient to the patient.

the right to advance notification if one's doctor cannot keep an appointment. The patient can refuse to see a substitute doctor and reschedule an appointment with the regular doctor.

the right to see any correspondence, articles, or conference materials concerning the patient.

the right to complain to any health service about infringements of any of these given rights.

D

Health Services

Community Health Department (Public Health)

The local health department is the official health agency for a particular city or county. Its duties include

safeguarding the purity of food and water;
promoting and providing inoculations for certain diseases;
communicable disease control;
control of mosquitoes, vermin, rats and other disease-carrying
   animals;
educating the public to health maintenance and disease control;
acting as a center for health information and education;
informing the public about new health developments and encouraging use of new services;
compiling health statistics;
relating local public health services to those of the state, and
   through the state agency to those of the U.S. Public Health
   Service, Department of Health, Education and Welfare.

HOSPITALS

There are different kinds of hospitals and they range in size from twenty-five beds to over a thousand beds. Some hospitals are operated primarily by governmental resources, some by religious organizations, some by private industry.

A *general community hospital* treats patients of all ages and with all kinds of sicknesses and medical conditions.

A *short-term hospital* treats only acute conditions that do not require a hospital stay lasting longer than about seven days.

A *long-term, or chronic care, hospital* treats patients with special long-lasting conditions such as tuberculosis or mental illness. Some of these are organized on an age basis.

A *medical center* is a grouping of hospitals that interrelate and share services.

A hospital provides such patient services as medicine, surgery, obstetrics, nursing, and rehabilitation. It may also maintain diagnostic, laboratory, dietary, health education, research, and professional training departments.

At the present time, a movement is underway to redefine and better utilize hospital space. The high cost of hospital care along with the high cost of improved instrumentation, research, and personnel is causing changes in the concept and practice of patient care. Some of these changes are

separate diagnostic centers rather than hosiptalization for tests.

separate treatment centers on a day-care basis that allow serving more patients per bed. For example, a patient may need only two days a week of hospital care. If that patient spends only eight hours a day for two days in a hospital bed, then the bed becomes available to care for at least two more patients a week on the same basis and either cuts down on the need to staff the nursing facility during the evening and night shifts or allows other patients to be served during those times.

increased home-care services to bring better medical, nursing, health education, and specific care training into the patient's home and thereby reduce the necessity for a long, costly, anxious hospital stay.

a better directing of patients into special care institutions such as short-term hospital rehabilitation training centers, short-term recovery nursing homes, chronic care homes, terminal care homes, etc.

Occupational Health

Many businesses offer services to protect and maintain the health of their employees. These include special safety measures in work that threatens health (such as coal mining), preventive health care through regular company-paid checkups, and insurance to cover unemployment resulting from work-related illness.

School Health

A school health service maintains a safe, healthy school environment and promotes and protects student health. Specific duties include

safety and sanitation in the classroom, laboratory, library, lunchroom, gymnasium, school building, grounds, and athletic fields;

preventing accidents and caring for emergencies;

checking on communicable diseases;

keeping health records on all students;

health education.

Voluntary Health Agencies

Health service agencies such as the American Cancer Society, the National Tuberculosis Association, and the American National Red Cross are supported by public contributions. These agencies identify and study specific health-related problems and advise on individual and public action. They also offer services that might otherwise be difficult to obtain because of newness or cost. They help in emergency situations and support professional education and research. A list of the main office of some national organizations is given in Appendix F. Other groups and local chapters are listed in the yellow pages of any telephone directory under "Social Service Organizations."

Health Machines

Many new kinds of work in health-related occupations have developed in recent years, some of which involves machines, such as:

Computers. Keep health records of patients for immediate referral, prompt and record the giving of treatments and medicines, etc.

Monitoring Consoles. Give continuous information on the physical status of patients — heartbeats, blood pressure, etc.

Automatic chemical analyzers. Perform as many as twenty different laboratory tests at one time and record the results on a strip chart.

Electronic devices. Scan X rays and enlarge, read, and convert them for storage and easy retrieval; send images by wire so that exact medical information and advice reaches remote areas.

Extracorporeal machines. Take over specific internal bodily functions. EXAMPLE: The kidney machine does the work of a kidney.

Other jobs relate to new or expanding fields of medical practice that require technicians, such as allergy environmentalists or genetic assistants.

Other Kinds of Available Health Care

Private doctor without a hospital affiliation. Takes care of office patients only. Patients requiring hospitalization are referred to doctors who specialize.

Private doctor with a hospital affiliation. Takes care of patients in the office and in the hospital. May or may not refer patients to specialists.

Private doctor with a hospital affiliation and an office in the hospital. From a health insurance patient's standpoint, there is a special advantage to using this doctor's services. Any diagnostic tests performed during an office visit are eligible for insurance coverage because they occur in a hospital.

Group practice. Several doctors who share one office and the care of all their patients.

Physician's assistant. A specially trained aide to a doctor who performs certain examinations, tests, and treatments.

Nurse practitioner, nurse midwife. Work together with physicians to perform certain functions once limited to doctors.

Emergency room treatment. A twenty-four-hour-a-day service by many government and private hospitals to take care of immediate problems requiring special equipment or treatment.

Outpatient clinic. A regular consultation and treatment service provided by many hospitals and available to anyone on a visiting basis and at a cost scaled to income.

Home Care. Medical and nursing services provided by a hospital or health agency in the patient's home.

Day-care hospital or center. Medical, nursing, and other professional services provided to patients who spend an entire day.

Nursing homes. Nursing and some medical and other professional services provided to those who live in the home. There are many specialty nursing homes, among them convalescent, chronic disease, terminal care, rehabilitation, geriatric, mental, alcoholic, drug addiction, and others.

Free clinic. Medical emergency care available without questions or fees to anyone in need. Operated through contributions of services, supplies, and money.

E

Doctors

All physicians are medical doctors, or M.D.s, but some specialize in a single area of patient care.

TITLE OF DOCTOR	SERVICE (MEDICAL ABBREVIATION)	FUNCTION
Allergist	Allergy	treats abnormal reactions to foods, pollens, dusts, and other substances
Anesthesiologist	Anesthesiology (Anesth)	gives anesthesia
Cardiologist	Cardiology (Card)	treats the heart and blood vessels
Dermatologist	Dermatology (Derm)	treats skin problems
General Practitioner	General Practice (GP)	treats all kinds of illnesses
Gerontologist, Geriatrician	Geriatrics	specializes in the care of geriatric patients
Gynecologist	Gynecology (GYN)	treats the female organs
Internist	Internal Medicine (Med)	treats adults with medical problems
Neurosurgeon, Neurologist	Neurology (Neuro)	treats the brain, spinal cord, and nervous system
Obstetrician	Obstetrics (OB)	cares for women during pregnancy, childbirth, and after delivery

TITLE OF DOCTOR	SERVICE (MEDICAL ABBREVIATION)	FUNCTION
Ophthalmologist	Ophthalmology (Eye)	treats the eye
Orthopedist	Orthopedics (Ortho)	treats muscles and bones
Otolaryngologist	Otolaryngology, or Ears, Nose, and Throat (ENT)	treats the ears, nose, and throat
Pathologist	Pathology (Path)	examines body tissues to aid in diagnosis or treatment
Pediatrician	Pediatrics (Ped)	treats children
Physiatrist	Rehabilitation (Rehab)	restores all possible body mobility after loss
Psychiatrist	Psychiatry (Psych)	treats mental disorders
Radiologist	Radiology (X ray)	works with radioactive tests and treatments
Surgeon	Surgery (Surg)	performs operations
Urologist	Urology (GU)	treats the male reproductive organs and the urinary organs of both sexes

F

National Organizations

That Furnish Information and Help with Health Maintenance

American Association for Health,
  Physical Education, and
  Recreation
1201 16th St., N.W.
Washington, D.C. 20036

American Association of Homes
  for the Aging
374 National Press Building
14th and F Sts., N.W.
Washington, D.C. 20004

American Association of Retired
  Persons
1225 Connecticut Ave., N.W.
Washington, D.C. 20036

American Association on Mental
  Deficiency
5201 Connecticut Ave., N.W.
Washington, D.C. 20015

American Cancer Society, Inc.
219 E. 42nd St.
New York, N.Y. 10017

American Congress of Rehabilitation Medicine
30 N. Michigan Ave.
Chicago, Ill. 60602

American Dental Association
211 E. Chicago Ave.
Chicago, Ill. 60611

American Diabetes Association,
  Inc.
18 E. 48th St.
New York, N.Y. 10017

American Foundation for the
  Blind, Inc.
15 West 16th St.
New York, N.Y. 10011

American Medical Association
535 N. Dearborn St.
Chicago, Ill. 60610

American Mothers Committee, Inc.
The Waldorf-Astoria, Room 2226
301 Park Ave.
New York, N.Y. 10022

The American National Red Cross
17th and D Sts., N.W.
Washington, D.C. 20006

American Nurses' Association, Inc.
10 Columbus Cir.
New York, N.Y. 10019

American Occupational Therapy
Association, Inc.
251 Park Ave. South
New York, N.Y. 10010

American Osteopathic Association
212 E. Ohio St.
Chicago, Ill. 60611

American Patients Association
1625 K St., N.W.
Washington, D.C. 20006

American Pharmaceutical
Association
2215 Constitution Ave., N.W.
Washington, D.C. 20037

American Physical Therapy
Association
1156 15th St., N.W.
Washington, D.C. 20005

American Podiatry Association
20 Chevy Chase Cir., N.W.
Washington, D.C. 20015

American Protestant Hospital
Association
840 N. Lake Shore Dr., Room 607
Chicago, Ill. 60611

American Psychiatric Association
1700 18th St., N.W.
Washington, D.C. 20009

American Psychological Association
1200 17th St., N.W.
Washington, D.C. 20036

American Public Health Association, Inc.
1015 18th St., N.W.
Washington, D.C. 20036

American Speech and Hearing
Association
9030 Old Georgetown Rd., N.W.
Washington, D.C. 20014

American Vocational Association,
Inc.
1510 H St., N.W.
Washington, D.C. 20005

The Arthritis Foundation
1212 Avenue of the Americas
New York, N.Y. 10036

Blue Cross Association
840 N. Lake Shore Dr.
Chicago, Ill. 60611

Consumer Federation of America
1012 14th St., N.W., Suite 402
Washington, D.C. 20005

Council of Jewish Federations and
Welfare Funds, Inc.
315 Park Ave. South
New York, N.Y. 10010

Council of Organizations Serving
the Deaf
4201 Connecticut Ave., N.W.
Washington, D.C. 20008

Council on Family Health
201 E. 42nd St.
New York, N.Y. 10017

Family Service Association of
America
44 E. 23rd St.
New York, N.Y. 10010

General Federation of Women's
Clubs
1734 N St., N.W.
Washington, D.C. 20036

League of United Latin American
Citizens
P.O. Box 896
Rancho Mirage, Calif. 92270

Mexican-American Opportunity
Foundation
2834 Whittier Blvd.
Los Angeles, Calif. 90023

National Association for Public
Continuing and Adult Education
1201 16th St., N.W.
Washington, D.C. 20036

National Association for the
Advancement of Colored People
1790 Broadway
New York, N.Y. 10019

National Association for the
Prevention of Addiction to
Narcotics
250 W. 57th St.
New York, N.Y. 10019

National Association for the
Prevention of Psychiatric
Hospitalization
c/o The Potomac Foundation for
Mental Health
5413 Cedar La.
Bethesda, Md. 20014

National Association of Blue
Shield Plans
211 E. Chicago Ave.
Chicago, Ill. 60611

The National Association of
Retail Druggists
1 E. Wacker Dr.
Chicago, Ill. 60601

National Cancer Foundation
1 Park Ave.
New York, N.Y. 10016

National Civil Liberties Clearing
House
3508 Albemarle St., N.W.
Washington, D.C. 20008

National Conference of Catholic
Charities
1346 Connecticut Ave., N.W.,
Suite 307
Washington, D.C. 20036

National Congress of American
Indians

1346 Connecticut Ave., N.W.,
Suite 312
Washington, D.C. 20036

National Council for Homemaker–
Home Health Aid Services, Inc.
1740 Broadway
New York, N.Y. 10019

National Council of Community
Mental Health Centers
2502 Belmont Blvd.   .
Nashville, Tenn. 37212

National Council of Health Care
Services
363 N St., S.W.
Washington, D.C. 20024

National Council on Alcoholism,
Inc.
2 Park Ave.
New York, N.Y. 10016

National Council on Family
Relations
1219 University Ave., S.E.
Minneapolis, Minn. 55414

The National Council on Hunger
and Malnutrition in the
United States
1000 Wisconsin Ave., N.W.
Washington, D.C. 20007

The National Council on the
Aging, Inc.
1828 L Street, N.W.
Suite 504
Washington, D.C. 20036

National Dairy Council
111 N. Canal St.
Chicago, Ill. 60606

National Dental Association, Inc.
P.O. Box 197
Charlottesville, Va. 22902

National Easter Seal Society for
Crippled Children and Adults
2023 W. Ogden Ave.
Chicago, Ill. 60612

National Federation of Licensed
Practical Nurses Incorporated
250 W. 57th St.
New York, N.Y. 10019

National Institutes on Rehabilitation and Health Services
1714 Massachusetts Ave., N.W.
Washington, D.C. 20036

National League for Nursing, Inc.
10 Columbus Cir.
New York, N.Y. 10019

National Legal Aid and Defender
Association
1155 E. 60th St.
Chicago, Ill. 60637

National Safety Council
425 N. Michigan Ave.
Chicago, Ill. 60611

National Therapeutic Recreation
Society
1700 Pennsylvania Ave., N.W.
Washington, D.C. 20006

Older Americans Resources and
Services Program

Duke University Medical Center
Box 3003
Durham, N.C. 27710

Pharmaceutical Manufacturers
Association
1155 15th St., N.W.
Washington, D.C. 20005

Psychiatric Outpatient Centers of
America
202 E. Bissell Ave.
Oil City, Pa. 16301

The Salvation Army
120 W. 14th St.
New York, N.Y. 10011

Sex Information and Education
Council of the U.S.
1855 Broadway
New York, N.Y. 10023

United Cerebral Palsy Association,
Inc.
66 E. 34th St.
New York, N.Y. 10016

The Volunteers of America
340 W. 85th St.
New York, N.Y. 10024

Index

Abduction, 46
Abortion, 345
Accident prevention. *See also* Safety
for geriatric patient, 246
Acetest (diabetes urine test), 237
Acetone, 236, 237
Activities
for geriatric patient, 205–206
of daily living. *See* ADL
for hospitalized child, 350
for sick child, 348
Acute heart disease symptoms
defined, 249
patient care, 249–250
Acute illness. *See also specific disease*
taking temperature in, 210
Adaptive equipment
for arthritic patient, 212
braces, 68–69
canes, 69–70
crutches, 71–74
custom-made, 64
feeding devices, 74–75
prostheses, 66–68
rules for use, 64–65
standard, 64
for stroke patient, 278
walkers, 75–76
wheelchairs, 76–79
Adduction, 46
Adenoids, 355

ADL (activities of daily living)
adaptive devices, 60–62
instructing patient, 60
for stroke patient, 272–274
testing and instruction, 59
ADL aids
for arthritic patient, 213, 214
for stroke patient, 273–276
Afterbirth, 337
Aggression in children, 264
Aging. *See* Geriatric patients
Alacta (infant formula), 327
Alcohol
cleaning with, 330
in geriatric diet, 209
infant navel care, 309
sponge bath, 190
Aliquots (portions), 179
Allergy(ies)
antihistamines and, 34
cause and care, 350
to infant formula, 326
to nonprescription medicine, 32
Amputation, 241
Anal itching, 356
Aneurysm, 248
Ankle
bandaging, 197
motions, 58
Antacids, 30–31
Antibiotics and antibacterials, 33–34

Anus, 170. *See also* Bowel and urine function
care in geriatric patient, 203
rectal suppository and, 38–39
Anxiety. *See also* Fears
heart symptom, 249
in children, 264
mental disorder symptom, 262
Aphasia, 277–278
Appendicitis, 187
Arm prosthesis, 67
Arm sling, 65–66
Arteriosclerosis, 248
Arthritis
bowel control, 213–214
equipment for treating, 211, 212–213
food and fluid, 213
footboard for, 116–117
medication for, 212
positioning of, 212
rehabilitation and physical therapy, 214
rest and, 212
Artificial replacements. *See also* Dentures; Prosthesis
removal after death, 227
Artificial respiration
mouth to mouth, 257–258
with respirator, 258–259
Asepsis, 191. *See also* Isolation techniques; Sterilization
Aspirin, 31
administering with milk, 212
arthritis medication, 212
Atrophy, 268
Axilla (armpit)
body temperature at, 21, 210

Backrest, 112
Back rub, 146
Bag of waters, 337
Bandages, 197. *See also* Dressings; Elastic bandages
Basins, sanitizing, 13
Bathing and grooming. *See also* Baths; Infant bathing
after death, 227
a blind patient, 230
doctor's orders for, 124, 133
evening care, 126–127
feet and nails, 144

genitalia, 208
geriatric patient, 208
hair care, 144, 148–154
importance of, 124–125
incontinent patients, 165
morning care, 125–126
reasons for, 128
safety, 11–12
shaving, 153–154
stroke patient, 275–276
supplies, 15
tooth care, 154–158
vaginal douche, 194–195
Bathroom care
cleaning and sanitizing, 13–14
in isolation technique, 220
Bathroom privileges. *See* BRP
Baths
after-bath care, 132
alcohol sponge bath, 190
arthritic pain, 214
assisting with bath or shower, 133–137
bicarbonate of soda, 221
complete bed bath, 128–131
arms and hands, 130
back and buttocks, 131
chest and abdomen, 130
equipment, 129
face, neck, and ears, 130
genitalia, 131, 138
legs and feet, 131
defined, 5
footbath, 137
paraffin, 185–186
partial bed bath, 132
sitz bath, 138–139
Bath thermometer, 310
checking heat treatment solutions, 180
Bed(s)
for arthritic patient, 211
bath. *See* Bathing and grooming; Baths
bed handy, 115
drawsheet, 14–15
during bowel and bladder function, 159, 161
dying patient, 226
heart disease patient, 250
hospital
electric, 116

Bed, hospital (*cont.*)
    fracture, 116
    handcrank, 115
    light for, 16
    protective sides, 115
    restraints, 118–119
    stroke patient, 268–269
    waste bag, 115
Bedboard, 113, 212, 244
Bedbugs, 117–118
Bedcradle, 115
Bedgowns, 18
Bedmaking
    equipment, 246
    fever-reducing bath, 310
    occupied bed, 120–121
    traction patient, 246
    unoccupied bed, 121–123
Bedpan and urinal
    bed position for, 161
    collecting specimens, 178–179
    disinfecting, 220
    equipment, 159–161
    helpless patient and, 161–162
    in isolation technique, 220
    offering, 159–161
        before meals, 84
    removal, 162
    sanitizing, 13
    vaginal douching, 194–195
Bedridden patients
    lifting and moving, 101
    mechanical lifting, 110
    positioning, 97
    pulling to sitting position, 103
    three-person carry, 111–112
    turning, 97
Bedroom care, 12–13
    in isolation technique, 220–221
Bedsores. *See also* Massaging;
        Positioning; Skin care
    bedding and clothing, 132–142
    decubitus ulcers, 142
    description, 142
    diabetic patient, 240
    patient care, 143–144
    pressure sores, 142
    skin breakdown, 7, 208
    stroke patient, 275
Bedtray, 114. *See also* Feeding
    isolation technique, 219

Behavior
    changes in sick child, 348
    in incontinence, 164
    infant, 337–338
    mentally disturbed patient, 263
    reactions to dying, 225–226
    stroke patient, 275
Benzine hexachloride, 153
Benzoin, tincture of, 173–174
Between-meal feedings, 91
Binders
    T-strap, 195–196
    uses of, 195
Birth. *See* Delivery
Birth canal, 337
Birth control, 282
Birthmarks, 350–351
Bladder. *See also* Urination; Urine
    childhood   toilet   training,   342,
        344
    infections in aging, 204
    irrigation, 169
Blankets. *See also* Electric blankets
        and pads
    infant, 315
Blindness and failing vision
    arranging   closets   and   drawers,
        231
    in children, 353
    eyeglass care, 233
    feeding patient, 231–232
    helpful organizations, 228
    legal definition, 228
    marking belongings, 230
    safety measures, 229
    social manners and, 232–233
    stroke patient, 267
    visual aids, 233
Blisters
    chicken pox, 221
    impetigo, 222
Blood
    chemistry and diet, 209
    circulation, 247
    clotting and Vitamin K, 285
    poisoning, 224
Blood pressure
    defined, 25
    diastolic, 26
    geriatric, 203
    hypertension, 248

Blood pressure (*cont.*)
  systolic, 26
  taking and recording, 26
Blood tests
  in diabetes, 241
  hospital nursery personnel, 285
  in pregnancy, 281
Blood vessel disease. *See* Heart disease
Body-arm hold for infants, 302–303
Body care. *See also* Skin
  after death, 227
Body trunk motions, 48–49
Body temperature
  alcohol sponge bath and, 190
  axillary, 21, 210
  changes in, 21
  conversion scale (Fahrenheit to Celsius), 210
  geriatric patient's, 210
  infant fever-reducing bath, 310
  oral, 21
  rectal, 21
  sick child, 348
  stroke patient, 269
Body weight
  aging patient, 210
  in heart disease, 251
  infant, 335–336, 340
    breast-fed, 321
    newborn, 311–312
  in pregnancy, 282
Boiling
  diapers, 318
  dishes, 14
  in sterilization, 14
Bones. *See also* Joints
  aging and, 202, 206
  fractures, 242–246
  infant skull, 298
Borax, for diaper care, 290, 318
Bottles, for infants. *See also* Infant feeding
  care of, 329–333
  Playtex nurser, 333
  preparation and filling, 333
Bowel and urine function. *See also* Enemas; Feces; Incontinence
  in aging, 203, 246

  in arthritis, 213
  bowel stimulants, 31
  cathartics, 31
  in colostomy care, 173–176
  constipation, 210, 351
  diarrhea medication, 33
  doctor's orders for, 6
  fecal impaction, 164
  geriatric diet and, 209
  hepatitis care and, 222
  in heart disease, 249
  incontinence, 164
  infancy and childhood, 340, 341
    breast-fed, 321
    constipation, 351
    diarrhea, 351
    formula-fed, 326
    newborn, 285, 337
    premature infant, 346
    training, 342, 344
  laxatives, 32
  liquid stools, measuring, 176
  stool specimen, 179
  in stroke patient, 267, 275
  in traction, 246
  urine specimen, 177, 179
Braces, 68–69
  in aging, 205
Brain damage and aging, 262
Brain disease, chronic, 262
Breads and cereals in diet, 83
Breast-feeding. *See* Infant feeding
Breast pump, 319
Breasts
  care in nursing mother, 323
  infant swelling, 354
  of newborn, 336
  in pregnancy, 281
Breathing. *See also* Respiration
  in aging, 204
  difficulty, 249
  noisy (in children), 354
  in respiratory system, 247–248
Bronchitis, 223
BRP (bathroom privileges), 133
Burns, bedcradle for, 114
Burping infant, 298, 329, 351, 353

Calories in diet, 94–96, 320
Canes, 69–70. *See also* Crutches
  for arthritis patient, 212

Cannula
  nasal oxygen, 255
Carbohydrates in diet, 80
Carbon dioxide
  in blood, 247
Cardiac monitor, 249
Cardiovascular blood vessel system, 247
Carriage
  infant safety, 294–295
  supplies, 287–288
Carrier of disease, 215
Cast. *See also* Traction
  application, 243
  patient care, 243–244
Cataracts, 204
Cathartics, 31–32. *See also* Laxatives
Catheter
  colostomy irrigation, 174–175
  doctor's orders, 168
  dying patient, 227
  fluid output, 177
  measuring drainage, 177
  nasal oxygen, 255
  urinary drainage, 268, 275
Cell growth and replacement, 201
Cerebral arteriosclerosis, 262
Cerebral palsy, 352
Cerebral vascular accident (CVA). *See* Stroke
Changes
  in aging patient, 203–204
  personality, 262
  skin color, 258
Charting. *See* Recording; *and specific illness*
Chemical sterilization, 191
Chicken pox, 221
Childbirth. *See* Delivery
Children. *See also* Infant care; Infant feeding; Infant handling
  caloric requirements, 320
  common health problems, 350–356
  group therapy, 265
  growth and development, 335–338
  mental disorders, 264
  nutrition, 319–320
  play therapy, 264–265

preparing for hospital stay, 349–350
  sick child care, 348–349
  tooth care, 156
  twins, 347
Cholesterol in diet, 93–94
Chronic disease(s)
  aging patient, 201, 203
  arthritis, 211–214
  diabetes, 236–241
  heart and lung disease, 251–260
  sick child, 349
Circulation
  bedsores. *See* Bedsores
  cast patient, 142
  elastic bandage, 196–197
  gangrene, 241
  geriatric patient, 203, 207
  respiratory system, 248
  stroke patient, 267
Circumcision, 285
  bathing infant, 308, 309
Cleft palate, 352
Clinitest for diabetes, 236, 237
Clorox, 14
Clothing
  chronic heart patient, 251
  diabetic patient, 240
  fracture first aid and, 242
  infant, 338. *See also* Diapers
    dressing, 314–315
    health and, 295
    laundry of, 291, 317–318
    premature, 346–347
    for twins, 348
  marking for blind patient, 230–231
  pajamas, changing, 105
  pinworms and, 356
  stroke patient, 276
  traction patient, 245
Clots (blood), 203
Coated tongue, 158
Coffee in diet, 209
Colds, common, 221
Cold treatments
  alcohol sponge bath, 190
  before applying, 187
  compresses, 188–189
  fever-reducing sponge bath, 310–311
  icebags, caps, and collars, 188

Cold treatments (*cont.*)
 soaks, 189–190
 uses of, 187
Colic in infants, 351
Colostomy
 bag, 173
 bulb syringe irrigation, 174–175
 changing unsterile dressing, 193–194
 douche bag irrigation, 174–175
Colostrum, 321, 337
Coma, diabetic, 240
Comfort and reassurance
 to a dying patient, 226
 to an incontinent patient, 164–165
Commode, 162–163
Communicable diseases. *See also specific disease*
 isolation technique, 215–216
 procedures, 217–221
 preventing spread of, 216
Communication problems
 aphasia, 277
 disturbed patient, 263–264
 geriatric patient, 206
 stroke patient, 277–278
Compresses
 hot, 183–184
 cold, 188–189
Condom urinary drainage, 169, 275
Condyloid joint, 42
Confused patient, 137
Congestion relief, 180
Conjunctivitis, 221–222
Constipation. *See also* Bowel and urine function; Fecal impaction; Toileting
 antacid use and, 31
 geriatric diet, 210
 infants, 351
Contagious disease, 215. *See also specific illness*
Containers for specimens, 178
Contamination, 215
Conversion scales
 ounces to cubic centimeters, 177
 pounds to ounces to kilograms, 312
 temperature from Fahrenheit to Celsius, 210

Cornstarch
 bath, 354
 chicken pox care, 221
Coronary care unit, 249
Coronary thrombosis, 248
Corsets, 70
 for traction patients, 245
Coughing, 204
Crab lice, 153
Cradle cap (infant), 351
Cradle hold for infants, 301–302
Crib (infant), 287, 294
Cross-leg hold for infants, 299–300
Croup, 351
Croup tent, 259
Crusts (catheter), 169
Crutches
 for arthritic patient, 212
 extension axillary, 71
 gaits with, 73
 Lofstrand or Canadian, 71
CVA. *See* Stroke
Cyanosis, 351

Dairy foods in diet, 83
Deafness. *See* Hearing loss
Death. *See also* Dying
 after-death care, 277
 in geriatric patients, 226
 legal forms, 226
Decubitis ulcers, 142, 143–144. *See also* Bedsores
 aging and, 203
Delivery
 hospital delivery room, 284
 Lamaze method of, 282
 packing for hospital, 283–284
 preparing for, 283
 sterile technique in, 191
Dehydration, 351–352
Denial, 225
Dental care. *See* Teeth; Tooth care
Dentures
 cleaning, 157–158
 geriatric digestive system and, 207, 209
 removal, 157, 227
Depression
 and arthritis patient, 211
 in children, 264
 emotional stage in dying, 225–226
 in geriatric patient, 206

Depression (*cont.*)
  as symptom of mental disorder, 262
Dextri-Maltose, 327
Diabetes
  antacid for, 31
  defined, 236
  diet, 238
  eye care and, 240
  footboard for, 116–117
  geriatric patient, 203, 209–241
  insulin therapy, 238–240
  nail care, 147
  patient identification, 240
  positioning patient, 240
  skin care, 240
  urine tests, 237
Diabetic coma, 240
Diabetic shock, 240
Diaper rash, 352
Diapers
  changing
    before and after feeding, 328–329
    equipment for, 316
    girls vs. boys, 316
    in sample routine, 339
  disposable, 288, 348
  for incontinent patient, 167
  laundering, 318
  numbers needed, 288
  pail for, 290, 291, 318
  premature baby, 346–347
  safety and, 295, 317
  twins, 348–349
Diarrhea, 176, 351. *See also* Bowel and urine function
  in infants, 338, 352
  medication, 33
Diastolic blood pressure, 26
Diet(s). *See also* Feeding
  for arthritic patient, 213
  bedtray for, 114
  daily requirements in, 83
  for diabetics, 238
  fluid balance and, 96
  for geriatric patients, 209–210
  for hepatitis patient, 222
  nutrition and, 81
  selection and preparation, 83
  special diets
    low-calorie, 94–95
    low-cholesterol, 93–94
    low-salt, 91–93
  standard diets
    bland, 89–90
    clear liquid, 87
    full liquid, 87
    regular, 90–91
    soft, 88
  types of, 6
Diet pills, 32
Diet sheet, 91
Digestive system
  aging and, 207
Disease. *See also specific name of illness*
  defined, 215
  and isolation technique, 215–216
Disinfectant
  for bedbugs, 117–118
  bleach or alcohol, 217
  bomb for fumigation, 221
  in isolation technique, 216
  for lice, 153
  pHisoHex soap, 216
Disposable
  bottles, 333–334
  binders, 196
  containers for postural drainage, 253
  diapers, 288
  gloves, 38, 166, 193, 194–195, 216, 217
  gowns, 217
  masks, 217
  nasal cannula, 255
  paper towels, 216, 217–218
  washcloths, 166
  wooden blades, 179
Disturbed patients
  bed restraints for, 118
  causes of, 261, 262–263
  children, 264
  home care of, 263
  symptoms of, 262
Diuretic medication, for heart patient, 251
Diverticulosis, 210
Dizziness, 249
Doctor(s)
  and patient's activity, 5
  arthritis patient, 213

Doctor(s) (cont.)
  binders and restraints, 195
  bowel and urine function, 6,
    164, 170
  diabetic patient, 236
  and geriatric patient, 205
  and hearing loss, 234
  heart disease, 248, 250
  inhalation therapy, 254
  paraffin bath, 185–186
  and patient's needs, 4–6
  postural drainage, 253
  pregnancy, 281–282
    reporting German measles,
      223
  and specimen collection, 178
  telephoning doctor
    in emergencies, 9
    when breathing stops, 257
    and vital signs, 5
Douche bag, for colostomy irriga-
    tion, 174
Douching
  during pregnancy, 282
  vaginal, 194–195
Drainage fluids, recording, 177
Drawsheet, 14–15, 104–105, 114–
    115
Dreaming, 291
Dressing(s), 195–196. See also
    Elastic bandages
  changing unsterile, 193–194
Drowning, 257
Dry heat. See Heat treatment;
    Sterilization
Dying. See also Death
  care of aging patient, 226
  description of, 226
  fear of, 202
  five emotional stages in, 225–
    226

Ear abscess, 223
Ear infection, 224
Ears. See also Hearing
  hold for treating child's, 303–
    304
  infant care, 307, 336
ECG. See Electrocardiogram
Eczema, 352
Edema, 251
EKG. See Electrocardiogram

Elastic bandages, 196–197
Elastic stockings, 197–198
Elbow motion, 53
Electrical equipment and O_2 tank,
    256
Electric blankets and pads, 181–
    182
Electric blender, 320
Electric heat lamps, 181
Electrocardiogram (EKG or ECG),
    248–249
Emergency procedures
  broken thermometer, 22
  when breathing stops, 257
Emesis, 176. See also Vomiting
Emotional development, infant,
    341
Emotional disorders, 261–263
  in children, 352
Emphysema, 252
Enema(s). See also Bedpan; Bowel
    and urine function; Toilet-
    ing
  for arthritis patient, 213
  for children, 351
  cleansing, 172–173
  defined, 170
  and fecal impaction, 164
  Fleet enema, 172–173
  and fluid balance, 96
  hold for infant, 301
  as internal heat treatment, 180
  mineral oil enema, 172–173
  rectal suppository technique, 39
  recording, 173
  soapsuds enema (SSE), 170–
    172
  stroke patient, 275
  tap water enema, 172
ENT specialist, 234
Euphoria, 353
Exercise(s). See also ADL (activi-
    ties of daily living)
  arthritis patient and, 214
  childbirth, 282
  body motion and, 43
  for geriatric patient, 207
  infant bathing and, 308
  for nursing mother, 323
  ROM exercises, 43–58
  therapy
    for handicapped children, 353

Exercise, therapy (*cont.*)
  for stroke patients, 269, 274–275
Exhalation (expiration), 248
Extension, 46
External heat treatment, 180–187
Eye care. *See also* Blindness and failing vision
  for diabetic patient, 240
  of infants, 307
  of newborn, 336
Eye congestion, 352
Eyeglass care, 233

False teeth. *See* Dentures
Fats, 81
Fears
  emotional disorders and, 261
  failing vision and, 228–229
  infant, 343
Fecal impaction, 172, 213
Feces, 38, 166
Feeding, 81–96. *See also* Diets; Infant feeding
  adaptive equipment for, 61
  between-meal nourishment, 91
  bedtray, 114
  blind patient, 231–232
  equipment, 74–75
  fluid intake in, 96
  helpless patient, 84
  isolation patients, 219
    giving liquids, 86
    giving solids, 86
  selection and preparation of foods, 83–86
  in stroke, 277
  whooping cough, 224
Feet care, 144
Fetus, 293, 319
Fever. *See* Body temperature
Fever-reducing bath, 310–311
Finger motions, 54
First aid
  artificial respiration, 257
  fracture, 242–243
  mouth-to-mouth resuscitation, 257–258
  telephoning doctor, 9
Fleet enema, 172–173
Flexion exercise, 46
Fluid balance, 96

Fluid intake
  geriatric traction patients, 246
  influenza and, 222
  measles and, 222–223
  scarlet fever and, 224
Fluid output, measuring, 176–177
Foley indwelling catheter, 168, 177, 275
Fontanelles, 308, 336
Food. *See* Diets; Feeding
Football hold for infant, 299
Footboard, 116–117
  for arthritis patient, 212
  design of, 116–117
  for dying patient, 226
Footprints, 284
Forceps, 192–193
Forearm motions, 53
Foreskin care, 309
Formula, infant. *See* Infant feeding, formula
Fracture
  cast application, 244–245
  compound, 242
  first aid, 242–243
  simple, 242
  traction, 245–246
  treatment, 243
Fruit in diet, 83
Fumigation, 221
Fungus infection(s)
  ringworm, 354
  thrush, 224

Gallstones, 203
Gangrene, 241
Garters, 198
General rules for treatment, 18–19
Genitalia. *See also* Bathing and grooming; Douching; Toileting
  catheter use and, 169
  cleaning and inspecting, 166, 169–170
  in condom drainage, 169–170, 275
  infant
    appearance in newborn, 337
    bathing, 309
    enlarged scrotum, 355
    vaginal bleeding, 355

Genitalia (*cont.*)
  sitz bath, 138–139
  washing, 131–138
Genital pads, 195–196
Geriatric patients
  activities and, 205
  blood circulation of, 207
  care of, 204–206
  cerebral arteriosclerosis, 262
  changing needs of, 206–210
  chronic diseases, 201
  constipation in, 172–210
  and diabetes, 241
  diet and feeding, 84, 209–210
  digestive system of, 207
  and dying, 226
  elastic bandages and, 196–197
  enemas and, 170–172
  fears of, 202
  fracture(s) of, 243, 246
  hair care of, 208
  heart disease in, 248
  hearing of, 208
  medical care goals for, 202
  mental disorders of, 262
  nervous system of, 207
  observing, 202–203
  physical therapy, 205
  process of aging, 201
  recording symptoms of, 203–204
  respiratory system of, 207
  sexual interest in, 204
  sight of, 2, 208–209, 230
  signs of aging in, 203–204, 246
  skin care for, 139, 208
  sleep and rest, 40, 209
  stroke and, 226
  temperature of, 210
  urinary system of, 208
  visual aids for, 233
German measles, 345
  in pregnancy, 223
Germicide, 219–220
Germs, 215
Glandular slowdown, 204
Glaucoma, 204
Gliding joint, 42
Gloves, sterile, 38, 166, 193, 194–
    195, 216, 217
Gowns, 18, 216, 217
Grief, 225–226

Group therapy, 265
Guide ropes for blind, 229

Hair care, 144
  combing snarled hair, 150
  geriatric patients, 204, 208
  infant, 336
  lice, 153
  shampoo, 148–149
    in bed, 150–152
    at sink, 152–153
Handicapped child, 352–353
Handling. *See also* Infant han-
    dling; Lifting and moving;
    Positioning
  general rules of, 97
Hands and feet
  paraffin bath, 185–186
Harelip, 352
Head and neck motions, 46
Head hold for children, 303
Hearing
  and child safety, 296
  of geriatric patient, 204, 208
  of newborn, 337
Hearing aid
  care of, 234–235
  for geriatric patient, 208
Hearing loss
  causes of, 234
  in children, 353
  protection for patients with, 235
Heart, defined, 247
Heart conditions
  in children, 352, 354
Heart disease. *See also* Oxygen
  acute
    care of patient with, 249–250
    diet for, 250
    oxygen for, 250
    positioning of patient, 250
    rest and, 249–250
    symptoms of, 249
  aging patient and, 248
  cardiac monitor and, 248
  chronic, 251
  common forms of, 248
    aneurysm, 248
    arteriosclerosis, 248
    attack, 248
    failure, 248
    hypertension and, 248

Heart disease (*cont.*)
  coronary care unit, 249
  electrocardiogram (EKG or
    ECG), 248–249
  respiratory system and, 248
  rheumatic fever and, 354
  medications
    diuretics, 251
    nitroglycerine, 251–252
    oxygen, 250, 252
Heat treatment
  for arthritic pain, 214
  external, 181
    compresses, 183
    soaks, 184–185
    towels, 185
    electric lamps, 181
    electric pads and blankets,
      181
    geriatric patient, 107
    hot water bag, 182
    hydrocollator steam pack,
      186–187
    paraffin bath, 185–186
  internal, 181
  medicinal heat, 180
  precautions, 182
Helpless patient, 112
  bedbath for, 128–132
  bedmaking, 121–123
  and brain damage, 262
  feeding, 84–85
  moving and handling, 96, 103–
    104, 109–112
  tooth and mouth care of, 158
  urinal and bedpan use, 161–162
Hemiplegia. *See* Stroke
Hemorrhoids, 203
  dressings, 193–194
Hepatitis, 216, 222
Hernia, 353
Hiccups, 353
High blood pressure, 248
Hinge joint, 42
Hip motion exercises, 56–57
Home care record or chart, 3, 6, 15
Hospital
  care of coronary patient, 249
  delivery of baby, 283–286
  preparing children for, 349–350
Hospital beds, 115–117
Hospital gowns, 216, 217

Host, 215
Hydrocollator
  pads, 214
  steam pack, 186–187
Hydrotherapy, 353
Hypertension, 209, 248

Ice bags, 188
Identification
  diabetic, 240
  hospital bracelets, 284
  of twins, 248
Immunity factors
  in colostrum, 321
Immunization shots, 338
Impetigo, 222
Incontinence. *See also* Bathing and
    grooming; Bowel and urine
    function; Toileting
  brain damage and, 262
  catheter use in, 168–170
  cleaning of patients, 165–166
  geriatric patient and, 204, 208
  nursing plan for, 165
  patients' reactions to, 164
  reassurance and, 164–165
  retraining and, 167
  T-strap binders, 195–196
  wheelchair and, 77
Incubator, 346
Infant bathing, 288, 292
  body-arm hold for, 302–303
  after circumcision, 308, 309
  cord care, 308–309
  equipment for, 289, 306
  face washing, 307
  fever-reducing sponge bath,
    310–311
  at four to six months, 341
  of newborn, 339
  procedures of, 306–308
  safety, 295
  sponge bath, 308–309
    genital care, 309
  tub bath, 306–308
  twins, 348
Infant care. *See also* Diapers; In-
    fant bathing; Infant feed-
    ing; Infant growth; Infant
    handling
  behavior, 336
  bowel function, 337, 340, 341

Infant care (*cont.*)
  burping, 239, 298
  circumcision, 285, 309
  clothing and dressing, 288–289, 314
    blanket wrapping in, 315
    diaper changing, 316–317
  common health problems, 350–356
  cord, 309, 336–337
  crying, 324, 337–338
  demand feeding, 324
  ear care, 307
  eye care, 307
  fever-reducing sponge bath, 310–311
  four-to-six-month-old, 343–344
  furniture for, 287
  genital care, 309
  handicapped child, 352–353
  height, 336, 340
  hospital and nursery care, 284–285
  laundering
    clothing and linen, 291, 317–318
    diapers, 288, 290, 317–318
    supplies for, 291
  measuring length, 311–312
  meconium, 337
  newborn, 335–339
  nostril care, 307
  pacifier, 325–338
  planning care, 291
  premature, 345–357
  rooming in (hospital), 286
  safety rules for, 293–296
  schedules in, 292–293, 339
  seven-to-twelve-month care, 343–344
  sick child, 348
  sucking and thumb sucking, 325, 340
  teething problems, 341
  three-month-old, 340–341
  toilet training, 344
  toy safety, 296–297
  twins, 347–348
  urination at three months, 340
  urine specimens, 317
  weighing, 311–312, 335–336
  whooping cough and, 224

Infant feeding
  breast-feeding, 285, 291, 295
    advantages, 321
    colostrum, 321, 337
    equipment for, 289–290
    expressing milk, 324
    formula feeding plus, 322
    infant bowel movements, 340
    mother's diet in, 322
    and nutrition, 319
    nipple care, 321–322
    offering the breast, 322
    scheduling, 321
    of twins, 347
  bottle care, 329–333
  burping, 239, 298
  cereal, 319, 325
  caloric requirements, 320
  commercially prepared foods, 319, 334, 342
  demand schedule, 324
  disposable bottles, 333–334
  equipment for, 290
  formula feeding, 284, 285, 289, 291, 325–334
    abbreviations, 327
    bottle care, 329–333
    breast-feeding and, 322
    burping, 239
    commercial preparations, 327, 334
    deciding on, 325–326
    Dextri-Maltose in, 327
    disposable bottles, 333–334
    doctor's orders and, 326–327
    equipment, 290
    formula order for, 327
    giving, 327–328
    infant safety, 295
    milks in, 327
    mixing with medicine, 349
    nipple flow, 328–329, 332
    reactions to, 326, 338
    scheduling of, 326
    sterile water in, 327
    sterilization methods, 329–333
    sugars in, 327, 332
    warming, 328, 329
  four-to-six-month-old, 341–342
  fresh food preparation, 319–320, 342

Infant feeding (*cont.*)
  newborn needs, 319
  nutrition and, 319
  premature infants, 346
  propping bottle, 338
  reaction to new foods, 342
  safety and, 295
  sucking, 325
  three-month-old, 341
  twins, 347–348
Infant growth
  during first year, 291
  newborn development, 335–338
    appearance, 336
    and breast-feeding, 321
    behavior, 337
    height, 336
    sensory development, 337
    weight, 311–312, 340
  premature development, 346–347
  at seven to twelve months, 342–343
    emotional development, 343
    habits, 343
    sensory development, 343
  at three months, 340–341
    appearance, 340–341
    emotional development, 341
    habits, 341
    height and weight, 340
Infant handling
  burping, 239, 298
  general rules for, 298
  lifting, turning, and holding, 298–305
  skull growth and, 298
  temperature hold, 301
Infection(s)
  common childhood, 350–356
  and geriatric diabetic, 241
  respiratory disease and, 252
  urinary, 168–169
Infectious diseases, 215
Inflammation. *See also* Bedsores
  arthritis, 211–214
  heat treatment for, 180
Inhalation (inspiration), 248
Inhalation therapy, 252, 254. *See also* Oxygen
  croup tent, 259

emergency shower technique, 260
  nasal cannula, 255
  nasal catheter, 255
  oxygen, 254–257
  safety rules for, 256–257
  respirator, 258–259
  steam inhalation, 259–260
Insomnia, 41
Insulin. *See also* Diabetes
  balance, 238
  coma and shock, 240
  defined, 236
  storage, 240
  urine testing and, 236–238
Insulin shock, 240
Internal heat treatment, 180
Interval nourishment, 91
Intravenous (IV) and fluid balance, 96
Iron tablets, 33
Irrigation
  bladder, with drainage tube, 169
  colostomy, 174–176
  vaginal, 194–195
Isolation technique
  communicable diseases and, 216, 221–224
  defined, 215
  equipment and room care in, 220–221
  feeding in, 219
  handwashing for, 217–218
  linen and laundry care, 219–220
  procedures of, 217
  respiratory disease and, 252
  setting up, 217
  waste disposal, 219
Itching (drug reaction), 33

Joints
  arthritis and, 211
  defined, 42
  of geriatric patient, 203
  ROM exercises for, 43–44

Karo syrup, 327
Kidney disease, 224
  footboard, 116–117
  swelling in limbs, 196
Knee motion exercise, 57
Knots, 119

Labeling, labels
in isolation technique, 217
of medicine, 30
of urine specimens, 178
Lactic acid, 145
Lactum (infant formula), 327
La Leche League, 324
Lamaze method (of childbirth), 282
Larynx, 247
Lateral position, 46
Laundering
baby bedding and clothing, 291, 317–318
bedding, 117
diapers, 288, 318
in isolation technique, 216, 219–220
twins' clothing, 348
Laxatives, 32
for heart disease patient, 249
for arthritis patient, 213
cathartics, 31–32
for nursing mother, 323
Legal forms, for dying patient, 226
Leg prosthesis, 67–68
Length of infant, 312
Lice, 153
Lifting and moving. See also Transfer
with drawsheet, 105–106
general rules, 101–104
of helpless patient, 103–104, 112
patient up in bed, 103
sitting position, 102
stance in, 101
three-person carry, 110–112
Lips. See also Mouth care
care of, 158
dying patient, 227
Loneliness, 261
Low-calorie diet, 94–95
Low-cholesterol diet, 93–94
Low-salt diet, 90–93, 209
Lung cancer, 252
Lungs, 247. See also Respiratory system

Magnifying glasses, 233
Marking system for blind patient, 230–231

Mask
in isolation technique, 216, 217
oxygen, 255
Massaging and oiling. See also Skin care
back rub, 146–147
forms of, 145–146
lotions and oils, 144–145
techniques, 146
Mattress. See also Beds
arthritis patient, 212
infant, 287
Meals. See Diet
Measles
German, 222–223
isolation technique, 215, 216
red or black, 223
Measuring fluid. See also Fluid balance
diuretics, 251
liquid stools, 176
Meat in diet, 83
Mechanical lifter, 109–110
Meconium, 337
Medicinal cold, 187
Medicinal heat, 180
Medicines and medications, 28–39
arthritis, 212
common prescription and non-prescription, 30–35
dosage and administration, 35–37
giving medicines at home, 37–38
geriatric diabetic patient, 241
government control of, 28
heart disease, 251–252
holds for administering to infant, 304–305
home care record, 6
mentally disturbed and, 263
mixing with food, 349
prescriptions, 29–30
rectal suppositories, 38–39
respirator delivery, 258
sick care box, 16
side effects, 28–29
storage, 16, 30
time sheets, 36
vaporizer delivery, 259
Menstrual period, 32, 281

Mental disorders
  care of, 263
  in children, 264–265
  emotional causes, 261
  physical causes, 262
  therapy, 264–265
Mental retardation, 352–353
Midline, 46
Milk
  for infant formula, 327
  in infant breasts, 354
  for nursing mother's diet, 323
Mineral oil
  enema, 164, 173
  laxative, 32
  in paraffin bath, 185–186
Minerals, 83
Miscarriage, 345
Moist heat, 191, 214. *See also* Heat
    treatment
Motion(s), 43. *See also* Physical
    therapy
  ROM exercises, 43–58
Mouth care. *See also* Teeth
  dying patient, 227
  helpless patient, 258
  infants, 308
  measles, 222–223
  thrush, 224
Mummy hold, 304–305
Mumps, 215, 216, 223
Muscular dystrophy, 352
Muteness in children, 353

Nail(s)
  cleaning for isolation technique,
    218
  color in chronic heart disease,
    251
Nail care, 144, 147–148
  impetigo, 222
  infant, 295
  stroke patient, 276
Narcotics, 34
Nasal cannula, 255
Nasal catheter, 255
Nervous system, 207
Neutral position, 46
Nevi. *See* Birthmarks
Newborn
  circumcision, 285
  delivery room care, 284

hospital needs, 284
identification bracelets, 284–285
nursery care, 285
rooming in, 286
Nipples
  breast, care in breast-feeding,
    285, 295
  disposable bottles, 333
  infant bottles, care of, 290, 295,
    330–333
  teething problems, 355
Nitroglycerine, 251–252
Nontoxic
  defined, 287
  toys, 297
Nose of newborn, 336
Numbness of fracture patient, 244
Nursery
  newborn care, 285
  personnel examination, 285
Nutrition. *See also* Feeding; Infant
    feeding
  necessary foods for, 83
  protein, carbohydrate, and fat
    requirements, 80–82, 276
  vitamins and minerals, 82–83

Obesity, 213
Observing
  rules for, 8–9, 203
  bowel function, 213
Occupational therapy, 17, 62
Olac (infant formula), 327
Olactum (infant formula), 327
OOB (out of bed), 133
Oral temperature, 21, 210
Organ transplants, 216
Osteoarthritis, 211
Oxygen (O_2)
  administering, 254–257
  cannula and, 255
  for cardiac patient, 252
  catheter or tube, 255
  for heart disease patient, 250
  mask, 255
  safety rules for, 256
  tank operation, 254–257
  tent, 254

Pacifiers for infants, 325, 338
Pain
  cast patient, 244
  chronic heart disease and, 251

Pain (*cont.*)
  as a symptom, 8
  relievers (medication), 34
Pajamas, changing, 105–106
Pancreas, 236
Paraffin bath, 185–186
Paralysis. *See* Stroke
Passive exercise, 44, 46
Patient care, 3–19
  activity and rest, 5
  cleaning and sanitizing unit, 12–14
  general rules for treatments, 18–19
  home care record, 6–7
  needs, 4–5
  observing, 7–8
  organizing, 16–18
  safety, 10–12
  sick care box, 14–16
  telephoning doctor, 9
Penis
  foreskin care, 169
  infant bathing, 309
Perineal care. *See* Genitalia
Phobia, 264
Physical therapy, 41–58. *See also* ADL (activities of daily living)
  aims of, 41
  arthritic patient, 214
  geriatric patient, 205
  program for, 42
  ROM exercises, 43–58
  stroke patient, 272
Pink eye. *See* Conjunctivitis
Pinworms, 356
Pivot joint, 42
Placenta, 337, 345–346
Plaque, 154
Plastic drawsheet, 13, 14–15, 104–105, 114–115
Play therapy, 264–265
Pneumonia, 223
Podiatrist, 147
Poisoning, 257
Positioning. *See also* Moving and lifting; Postural drainage
  arthritic patient, 212
  cast patient, 244
  in chair, 99

chronic heart patient, 253
diabetic patient, 240
with drawsheets, 104
dying patient, 227
geriatric traction patient, 246
heart patient with acute symptoms, 250
infant, 338, 341
after ROM exercises, 99
stroke patient, 269–272
supports, 99
wheelchair, 79
Postural drainage, 252–253
Potassium in diet, 209
Pregnancy. *See also* Delivery
  doctor and, 281–282
  German measles and, 223
  length of, 345
  signs of, 281
  unusual conditions of, 345–346
Premature
  delivery, 345
  infant care, 345–347
Prescriptions (medication), 29–30
Pressure points, 245
Pressure sores. *See* Bedsores
Prestroke symptoms, 267
Prickly heat, 354
Prone position, 46
Propping (infant feeding), 338
Prostate trouble, 204
Prosthesis
  arm, 67
  defined, 66
  leg, 67–68
  skin care and, 67
  wheelchair use with, 76
Protective (bed) sides, 114
Protein in diet, 81, 209, 276
Psychiatrist, 264
Psychological needs
  aging patient, 202
  incontinent patient, 164–165
Psychological treatment for handicapped child, 353
Pulse rate
  heart disease, 249
  normal, 23
  recording, 24
  scheduling, 5
  taking, 24

Range of motion exercises. *See* ROM
Recording (charting)
  diabetic diet, 238
  enemas, 173
  fluid intake, 96
  fluid output, 176–177
  geriatric symptoms, 203–204
  home care record, 6–7
· infant
    reaction to formula, 338
    weight, 311–312
  medications
    sick child, 348–349
  specimens
    stool, 179
    urine, 178–179, 236, 237–238
Recreation activities, 15, 17, 205–206, 350
Recreational therapy, 62–63, 353. *See also* ADL (activities of daily living)
Rectal
  body temperature, 21
  suppository medication, 38–39
Reduction for fractures, 243
Rehabilitation
  arthritis patient, 214
  stroke patient, 272–273
Relaxing comfort measures, 41, 145
REM sleep, 40
Respiration. *See also* Respiratory system
  artificial, 257
  counting, 24
  defined, 24
  noisy breathing in children, 354
  with respirator, 258
Respirator
  administering, 258
  fears of patient, 259
  skin care, 258
Respiratory disease
  kinds of, 252
  respirator, 258
  treatments
    artificial respiration, 257–258
    drainage, 253
    inhalation, 254
    steam, 259–260

Respiratory system, 247–248
  geriatric patient, 207
Rest and sleep
  arthritis patient, 212
  geriatric patient, 40, 204, 209
  heart disease patient, 249
  infant needs, 291–292, 339, 341, 343–344
  insomnia, 41
  nursing mother, 323
  premature baby, 346–347
  REM sleep, 40
  sick child, 348
Restraining hold for child, 304–305
Restraints, 195–196
  directions for, 118
  equipment, 119
  knots, 119
Resuscitation, 257
Rheumatic fever, 224, 354
Rheumatoid arthritis, 211. *See also* Arthritis
Right to die (legal forms), 226
Ringworm, 354
ROM (range of motion) exercises, 43–58
  ankle motions, 58
  arthritic patient, 214
  body trunk motions, 48–49
  elbow motions, 52–53
  finger motions, 54
  forearm motions, 53
  head and neck motions, 47
  hip motions, 56–57
  knee motions, 57
  shoulder motions, 50–51
  stroke patient and, 269–272
  thumb motions, 55
  toe motions, 58
  wrist motions, 54
Room care
  cleaning, 12–13
  isolation technique, 217, 219, 220
  organizing, 16–17
  safety, 11
  sanitizing, 13
  stroke patient, 269
Rooming in, 284, 286
Rotation exercise, 46

Saccharin, 238
Safety
  accident prevention, 10
  adaptive devices, 64–65
  bathroom, 11
  bed, 10
  bedroom, 11
  blind patient, 229–230
  clothing and walking equipment, 11
  food, 12
  geriatric patient, 206, 209
  hallway and stairs, 11
  infant and child care, 293–296
    toy safety, 297
  oxygen, 250, 256
  positioning equipment, 107
  special measures, 10–11
Salt
  in diet, 91–93, 209, 250
  substitutes, 93
Sanitary napkin
  with rectal suppository, 39
Sanitizing. See also Sterilization
  basins and plastic, 13
  bathroom, 13
  bedding, 14
  bedroom, 12
  toileting equipment, 13
Scales, baby, 311–312
Scrotum, in infant, 355
Self-care of patient
  ADL programs in, 59–60
  dressing and undressing, 60–61
  eating, 61, 74–75
  geriatric patient, 204
  mobility, 61–62
  moving about in bed, 60
  personal grooming, 60
  stroke patient, 272–274
  using the hands, 61
Senile brain disease, 262
Sensory development in infants, 337, 341
Sexual interest
  geriatric patient, 204
Shaving
  geriatric patients, 208
  grooming male patients, 153–154
  stroke patient, 276
Sheepskin, for bedsores, 143

Sheets
  bedmaking, 117, 120–123
  with electric pad and blanket, 181
  infant crib and carriage, 289
  mummy hold for child, 304–305
Shiatsu massage, 145–146
Short leg brace, 68–69
Shoulder motion exercises, 50–52
Shower. See also Bathing and grooming
  assisting with, 133–137
  emergency steam inhalation, 260
  stroke patient, 275
Sick care box, 14–16
Sight. See also Blindness and failing vision
  aging and, 204, 206
  in newborn, 337
Simulac (infant formula), 327
Single T-binder, 195–196
Sitz bath, 138–139
Skin. See also specific condition
  appearance in newborn, 337
  changes in aging patient, 204
  color
    cast patient, 244
    heart disease, 249, 251
    premature infant, 346
    traction patient, 245
  observing, 140–143
Skin care. See also Bathing and grooming; and specific condition
  aging and, 139
  bedding and clothing, 142–143
  bedsores, 143–144
  body alignment, 143
  bowel function and, 140
  colostomies, 173
  components of, 139–140
  crutch use, 74
  decubitus ulcers, 143–144
  diabetic, 240
  diet, 140
  eczema, 352
  fracture, cast, and traction patient, 244–246
  geriatric patient, 208
  heat lamp and, 181
  massaging and oiling, 144–145

Skin care (*cont.*)
  physical activity and, 140
  respirator and, 258
  stroke patient, 275
Skull, of newborn, 298, 336
Sleep. *See* Rest and sleep
* Slings, arm, 213
Smell
  newborn, 337
  observing patient symptoms, 8
Smoking
  lung cancer, 252
  oxygen tank safety, 256
Soaks
  cold, 189–190
  hot, 184–185
Soapsuds enema (SSE), 170–172
Social manners for home care
  blind patient, 232–233
  hearing loss patient, 235
  incontinent patient, 164–165
  mentally disturbed patient, 263
Special clothing
  traction patient, 245
Specimens
  defined, 177
  infant, 317
  stool, 179
  urine, 178–179
Speech. *See also* Communication
    problems
  geriatric patient, 203
  stroke patient, 277–278
Sperm strength and adult mumps,
    223
Sphygmomanometer, 26
Spinal bones, 42
Splint
  first aid for fracture, 242–243
Sputum cup, 207, 252, 259
SSE. *See* Soapsuds enema
Steam
  emergency shower technique,
    260
  inhalation therapy, 259
  packs, hydrocollator, 186–187
Sterile techniques (asepsis), 191–
    193
Sterile water. *See also* Mouth care
  infant bathing, 306–309
  infant formula, 327

sick child care, 348
thrush infection, 224
Sterilization
  bedpans and urinals, 13
  diapers, 318
  dishes, 14
  general rules of, 192
  infant formula, 329–333
  isolation equipment, 220–221
  methods of, 191
  techniques, 191–193
  waste, 14
Stethoscope, 26
Stoma. *See* Colostomy
Stool. *See also* Bowel and urine
    function; Specimens
  examination for hospital person-
    nel, 285
  pinworms, 356
Strep throat, 223–224
Stroke
  adaptive equipment, 278
  ADL bath aids, 275–276
  ADL rehabilitation, 272–273
  bathing and grooming, 275–276
  bowel control, 267, 275
  care area, 268–269
  causes of, 266
  communicating, 277
  CVA defined, 266
  dressing, 276
  exercises, 274–275
  food and fluid, 277
  footboard, 116–117
  hemiplegia, 267–268
  nail care, 276
  positioning, 269–272
  prestroke symptoms, 267
  ROM exercises, 269–272
  shaving, 276
  skin care, 275
  stages in, 268
  visual problems, 267
  vital signs, 269
Stump sock, 67–68
Sucking in infants, 321, 325
Sugar(s)
  in diabetic diet, 238
  infant formula, 327, 332
  substitutes, 238
Supine position, 46
Suppositories, 39, 164

Surgery for fracture patient, 243, 245
Surgical collars, 245
Sweat, measuring, 176
Sweating and aspirins, 212
Swedish massage, 145
Symptom(s). *See also specific topic*
  changes in, 8
  defined, 7
  describing, 7–9
  pain and, 8
Systolic blood pressure, 26

Tank. *See* Oxygen
Teeth. *See also* Mouth care
  children, 157
  cleaning, 155–156
  dentist, 156
  dentures, 157–158
  diabetic patient, 241
  diet and, 155, 209–210
  equipment, 157
  geriatric patient, 203, 207
  tartar, 154
Teething problems (infant), 355
Telephoning doctor, 9, 257
Temperature. *See also* Body temperature
  bath and bathroom, 134–135
  infant bath, 306, 310
  infant formula, 328–329
  shower, 133, 135
Temperature hold for infants, 301
Tetanus, 216
Therapy. *See* ADL; Occupational therapy; Physical therapy; Recreational therapy
Thermometers. *See also* Body temperature
  axillary temperature, 21
  breakage, 22
  infant, 310
    temperature hold, 301
  oral, 21
  reading, 22
  rectal, 21
Throat cultures, 285
Thrush, 224
Thumb motion exercise, 55
Thumb sucking, 325
Tincture of benzoin, 173–174

Tingling, 244
Toe motion exercise, 58
Toileting. *See also* Bedpan and urinal; Bowel and urine function; Urination
  ADL devices, 60
  equipment
    bedpan and urinal, 159–162
    commode, 162–163
    grab bars, 162
  incontinent patient, 60, 167
  isolation technique, 220
  sanitizing, 13–14
  specimens, 177–179
  storage, 15
Toilet training, 342, 344
Tongue-tie of children, 355
Tonsillitis, 355
Touch(ing)
  mentally disturbed patient, 263
  newborn sense of, 337
  patient well-being, 144
Trachea, 247
Traction, 116
  beds for, 116, 246
  defined, 243, 245
  elastic, 245
  geriatric patient, 246
  positioning, 245
  skeletal, 245
  skin care, 245
  special clothing, 245
  weights, 245
Tranquilizers, 35
Transfer of patients
  from bed, 107–109
  mechanical lifter, 109–110
  three-person carry, 110–111
Trapeze in traction, 245
Tray. *See* Feeding
Treatment. *See also specific illness*
  cold, 187–190
  fracture patient, 243–245
  general rules, 18–19
  heart and lung disease patient, 248–249
  heat, 180–187
  mentally disturbed patient, 263
    children, 264–265
  recording in chart, 15
Trembling, 203

Tub baths. *See* Bathing and grooming
Tube
  catheter drainage, 168–170
  oxygen (O_2), 255
Tuberculosis, 216, 252
Turning. *See also* Positioning
  in bedmaking, 120
  bedridden patient, 96
  infant, 338, 341
  patient self-help, 106
  stroke patient, 269–272
Twins, 347–348. *See also* Infant care

Ulcers, decubitus. *See* Decubitus ulcers
Umbilical cord, 284, 336–337
  infant bathing, 308, 309
Umbilicus, hernia in, 352
Unsterile dressing, 193–194
Urinal, offering before meals, 84, 159–161. *See also* Bedpan and urinal
Urinary catheter
  drainage, 168
  dying patient, 227
Urinary condom
  drainage, 168, 169–170
Urinary system. *See also* Urination; Urine
  geriatric patient, 208
  infection, 168–169
Urination
  cast patient, 244
  diuretics and, 251
  dying patient, 227
  geriatric patient, 204, 208
  helpless patient, 161–162
  incontinent patient, 164–167
  infant, 285, 340
  measuring, 176–177
  in morning, 125
  during pregnancy, 281
  stimulating, 162
  with urinal, 159–161
Urine
  fluid balance, 96
  infant specimen, 311
  measuring output, 96, 176–177
  newborn, 285

specimens, 177–179
  tests, in diabetes, 236–238
Uterus, 293, 337, 345–346

Vaginal
  bleeding, in infants, 355
  douching (irrigation), 194–195
    in pregnancy, 282
  dressing, 193–194
  inflammation, 32
Vaporizer therapy, 259
Varicose veins, 203, 241
Vision. *See* Blindness and failing vision
Vital signs
  defined, 5
  recording in home care chart, 6
  stroke patient, 269
  taking, 20–27
Vitamin A, 32, 82
Vitamin B, 32, 82
Vitamin C, 33, 82
Vitamin D, 32, 82
Vitamin E, 82
Vitamin K, 82, 285
Vitamins in diet, 82, 209
Voice box, 247
Vomiting (emesis)
  in infants, 338
  measuring fluid output, 176
Vulva, infant, 309

Walkers, 76
  arthritis patient, 212
  geriatric patient, 205
Washing
  hands in isolation technique, 216, 217–218
  clothing. *See* Laundering
  infants. *See* Infant bathing
  patients. *See* Bathing and grooming
Waste disposal
  burning, 14
  in incontinence, 165–166
  in isolation technique, 219
Water
  in diet, 83
  enemas, 170
  fluid balance, 96

Water (*cont.*)
  hiccup care, 353
  infant with immunization shots,
    338
Weight. *See* Body weight
Weights
  conversion scales for, 177, 312
  traction, 245
Wheelchair, 76–79
  arthritis patient, 212

bedsores, 144
geriatric patient, 205
grab bars, 163
toileting, 77, 173
Wheezing, 251
Whooping cough, 224
Windpipe, 247
Wintergreen, 180
Worms, 356
Wound infection, 216